The Book on Time

AN OWNER'S MANUAL
FOR THE TIME OF YOUR LIFE

BY ETHAN HAWKES
CO-FOUNDER OF

bernard & hawkes

Table of Contents

If life came with an owner's manual,
would you take the time to read it?

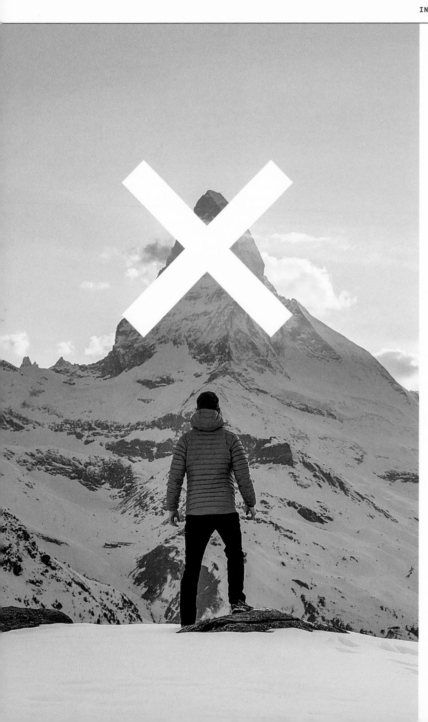

I'VE YET TO MEET the person who won at life—someone who completely and undeniably beat everyone else. This either means that I need to get out more or that life isn't all about reaching one predefined destination. The beauty and complexity of life seems to be in the wide range of options on where to go, how to get there, and whether you'll like where you end up—or enjoy the journey.

The catch is, we only have so much time. Without this almost invisible constraint, we could explore every possible path. Time is what forces us to constantly make choices that require small and large trade-offs. It is these choices that reveal what we value and ultimately determine the type of life we have. In other words, what defines who we are and who we will become is how we choose to spend our time.

Many of us live as if we're too busy to slow down and think about why we're spending our time the way we do. For too long I lived this way and often still do. Early in life, our parents guide us, then school keeps us busy, then we prirotize career demands, and then we may have a family to support. We may reach the end and wonder if we were the driver or passenger in our own lives. Getting a grip on ways to invest time well is a lot like finding the steering wheel.

This manual isn't about how to win at life. It's mostly about how not to lose—by learning from other people with more accumulated life experience, recognizing with humility that we don't have enough time and don't want to learn the painful lessons firsthand. Nor do we want to waste time reinventing the wheel in order to learn what reliably works.

This manual is about gaining an appreciation for time and learning how to make better decisions about it in our lives. It's ultimately about trying to avoid one risk in life that we never want to take—that someday we'll look back on life with deep regrets.

I've been told that life is long enough if you live it well. And that's about as close to winning as it gets.

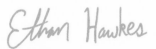

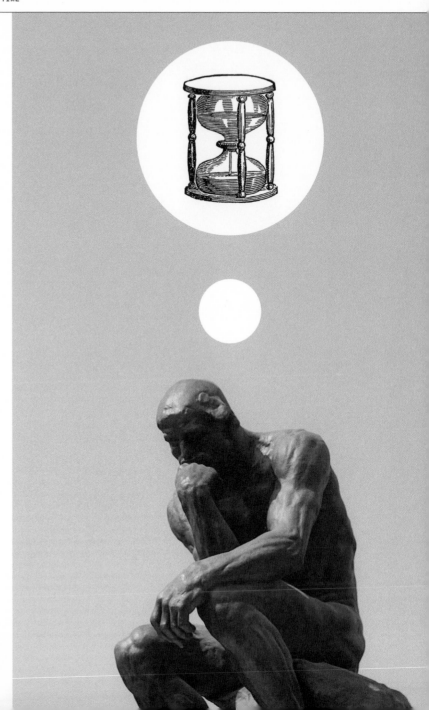

Here's the big reveal:

(spoiler alert)

Time well spent leads to a life well lived.

So, how can you invest your time wisely and live well?

Let's find out.

To get started on the search for answers, our team of Harvard-educated researchers went through the latest scientific findings from over 250 peer-reviewed studies on topics ranging from astrobiology to the gut microbiome to life regrets. We also brushed up on ~3,000 years of philosophy until our eyes glazed over.

Even with the benefit of this research, we found that a surprising amount of insight and the most helpful frameworks came from simply taking the time to think things through from the foundational principles. Consider this manual a baton that we are now passing to you in the hopes that it enhances your own thinking and journey through time.

This 180-page owner's manual should take you about **48 minutes** to skim (and a lifetime to master).

In return you will receive:

- A deeper understanding and appreciation of time
- Insight on how we spend our time and why
- Guidance on how to avoid common pitfalls
- The best thinking based on scientific research, philosophy, and ancient wisdom
- Actionable ways to prioritize and make the most of your time
- Pointers that will help you think through the important questions and decisions for yourself

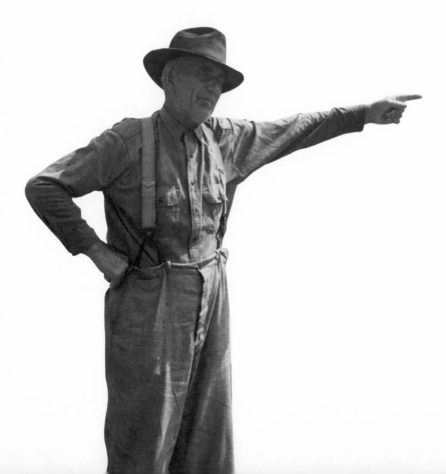

Time's a wasting.
Onward.

PART ONE

What time is it—and how much do we have?

Understanding Our Relationship to Time

We measure time circularly.

For almost all of human history, people were acutely aware of changes in the weather. By far, the most significant changes were driven by planetary movements.

As a result, the calendar and ways of measuring time are centered on these cycles including years (orbits of the Earth around the Sun), months (orbits of the moon around the Earth), and days (rotations of the Earth).

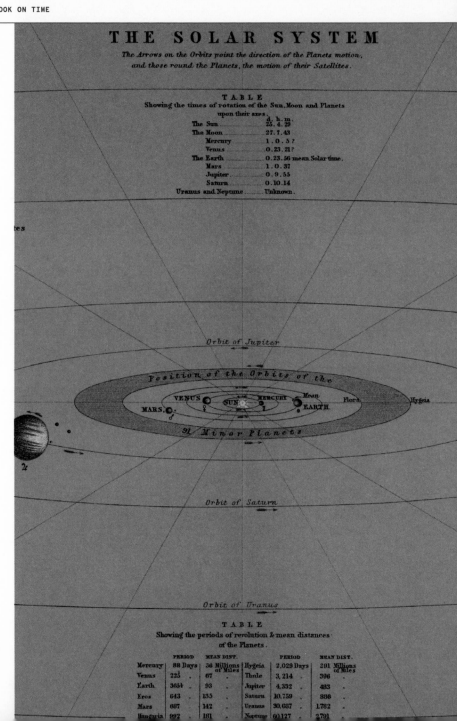

We experience time linearly.

——

We naturally split time into the past (things that were), present (things that are), and future (things that are yet to be).

No one can agree on precisely what moment is the present versus the past or future, but we generally experience some window of time as being now.

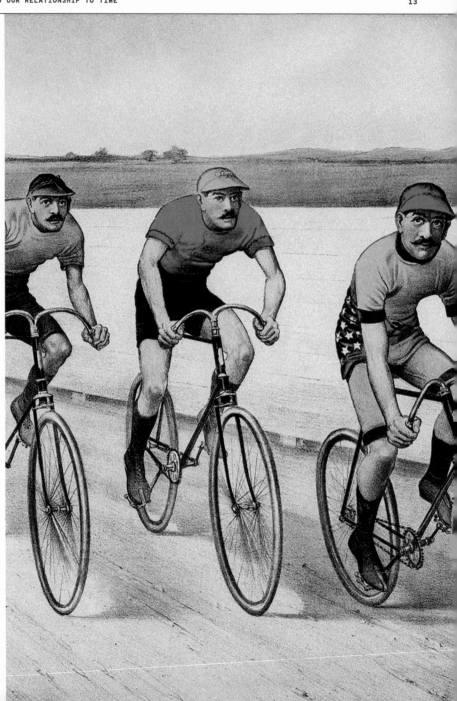

Turns out it's all relative.

———

After Einstein published the Theory of Relativity in 1905, physiscists realized that our ancestors pretty much had it all wrong.

Turns out that time isn't constant, that there is no universal present, and that a host of other head-scratching implications still need to be resolved.

For better or worse, the more extreme effects only really apply in noticeable amounts at far greater distances and speeds than we are likely to experience.

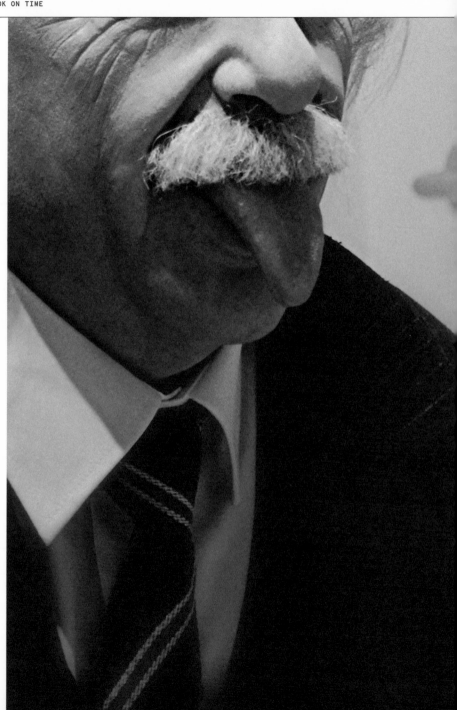

Any way you look at it, time has been around quite a while. Even though we haven't.

Everything we know about humans from the caveman to current day

Life on Earth

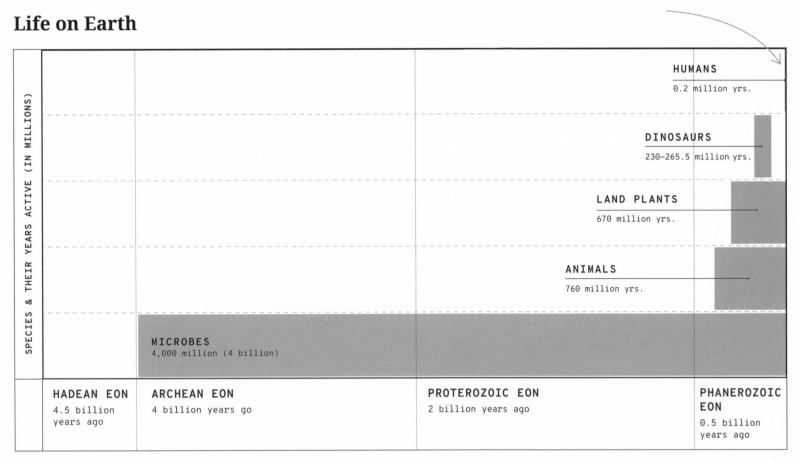

SPECIES & THEIR YEARS ACTIVE (IN MILLIONS)

HUMANS
0.2 million yrs.

DINOSAURS
230–265.5 million yrs.

LAND PLANTS
670 million yrs.

ANIMALS
760 million yrs.

MICROBES
4,000 million (4 billion)

HADEAN EON	**ARCHEAN EON**	**PROTEROZOIC EON**	**PHANEROZOIC EON**
4.5 billion years ago	4 billion years go	2 billion years ago	0.5 billion years ago

Source: "Timeline and History of Life." Wikipedia and Journal of Astrobiology

But within that sliver of time,
we've left a massive impact.

We're multiplying exponentially.

World Population (10,000 BCE — 2020)

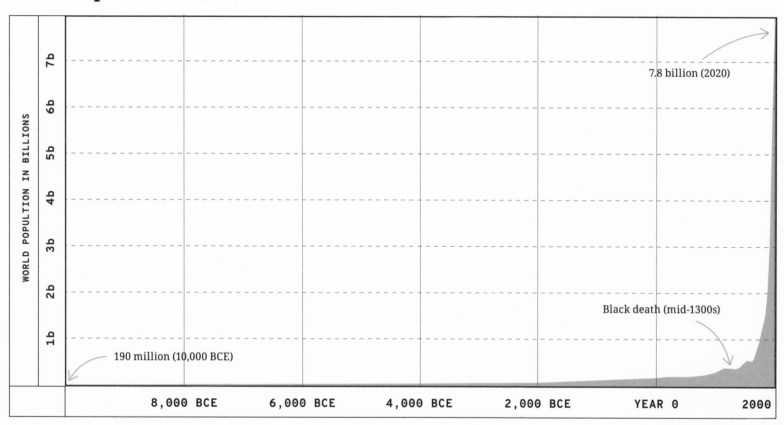

Source: "World Population Growth." OurWorldinData.org

We're consuming and producing more and more.

Gross Domestic Product Per Person, Globally (1870 — 2016)

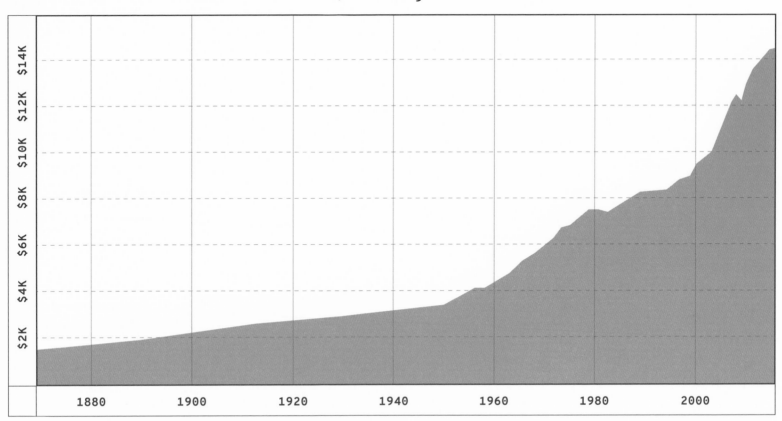

Source: "World GDP per Capital." OurWorldinData.org, Maddison Project Database (2018)

And we're all living longer.

Global Life Expectancy (1770 — 2015)

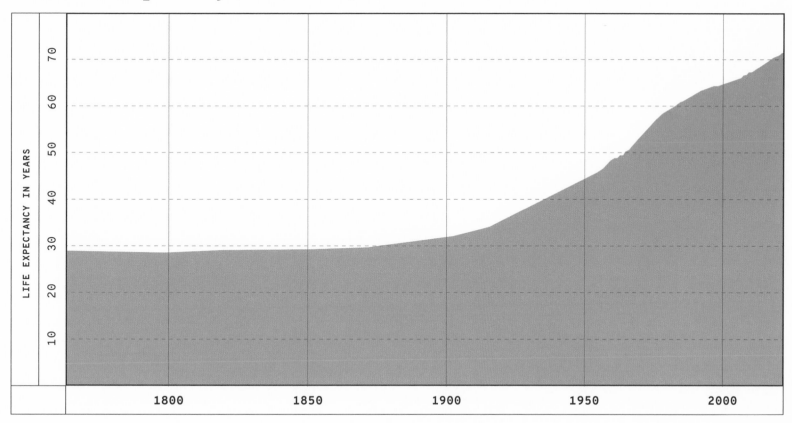

Source: "Life expectancy." OurWorldinData.org, UN Population Division (2019)

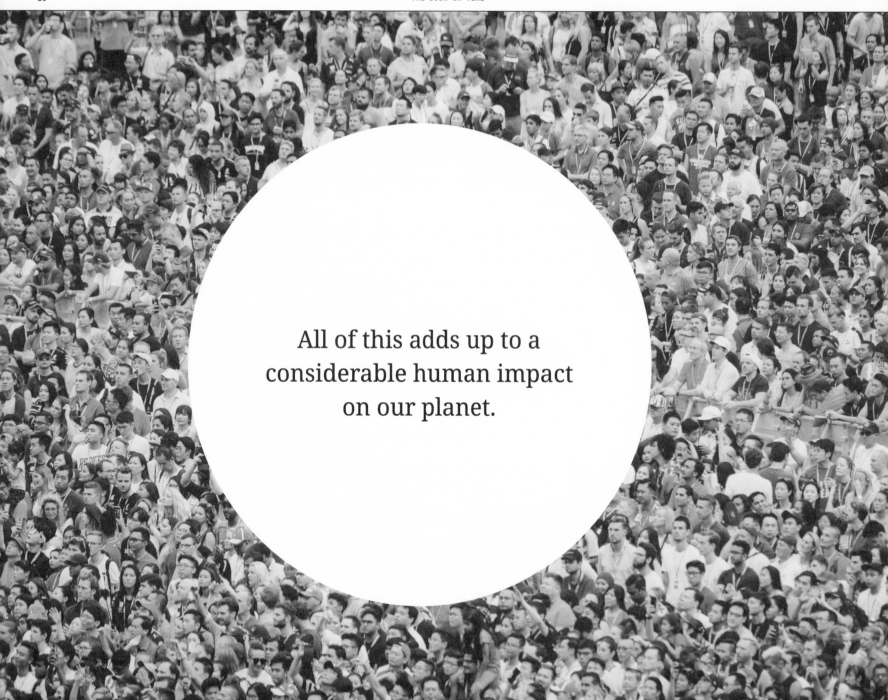

All of this adds up to a
considerable human impact
on our planet.

Most other species haven't fared as well as we have.

Animal populations fell by 68% in the past 50 years according to World Wildlife Fund studies of mammals, birds, fish, reptiles, and amphibian species.

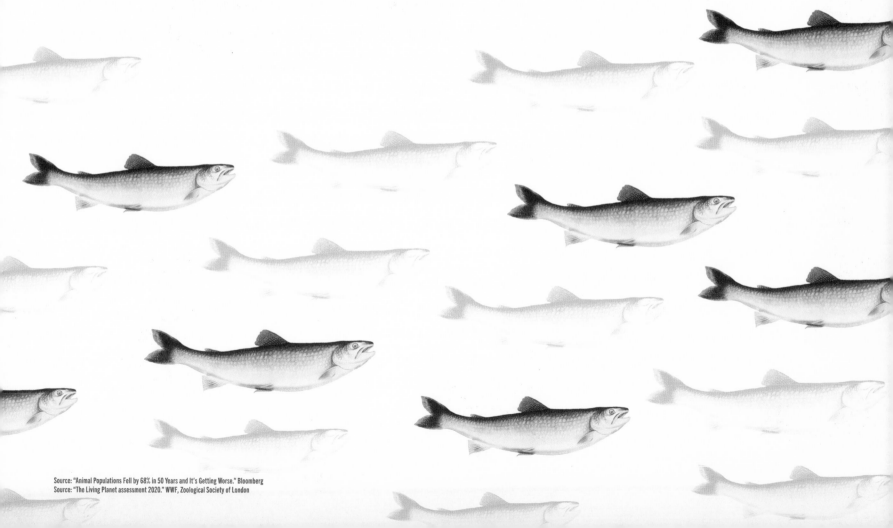

Source: "Animal Populations Fell by 68% in 50 Years and It's Getting Worse." Bloomberg
Source: "The Living Planet assessment 2020." WWF, Zoological Society of London

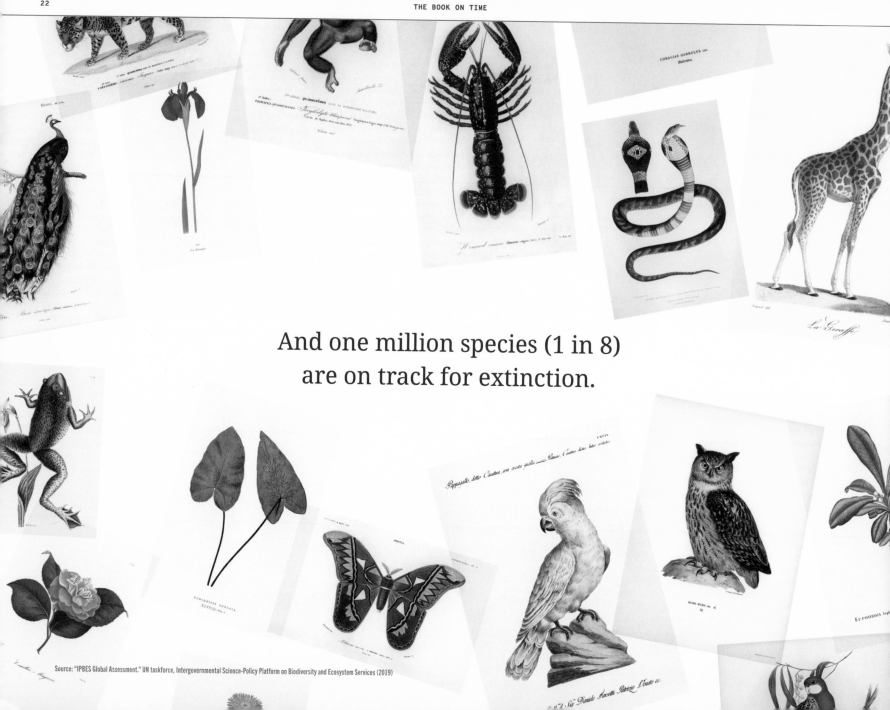

And one million species (1 in 8)
are on track for extinction.

Source: "IPBES Global Assessment." UN taskforce, Intergovernmental Science-Policy Platform on Biodiversity and Ecosystem Services (2019)

To be frank, humans may not fare well either.
Problems are likely brewing for future generations.

———

Our economy and way of life are built on continued growth. Otherwise, our economic system becomes unstable, like a bicycle losing speed. Anything constantly growing is by definition growing exponentially.

From a biology and math perspective, continued exponential growth is incompatible with a finite host environment—be that a petri dish, organism, island, or world.

Maybe this time is different. We don't know yet what the carrying capacity of our planet is. If the resource side is finite, four key factors determine long-term sustainability:

- Population size and growth rate
- Level and type of economic production and consumption
- Technological progress, with the potential to both accelerate and mitigate our impact
- Our commitment to getting along with one another and stewarding the planet's resources

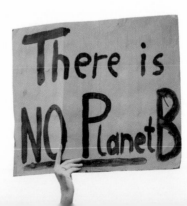

But before we get too bummed out, let's remember:
we're still here.

Most people who have ever lived are no longer with us.
Their time on Earth has ended. Yours has not (yet).

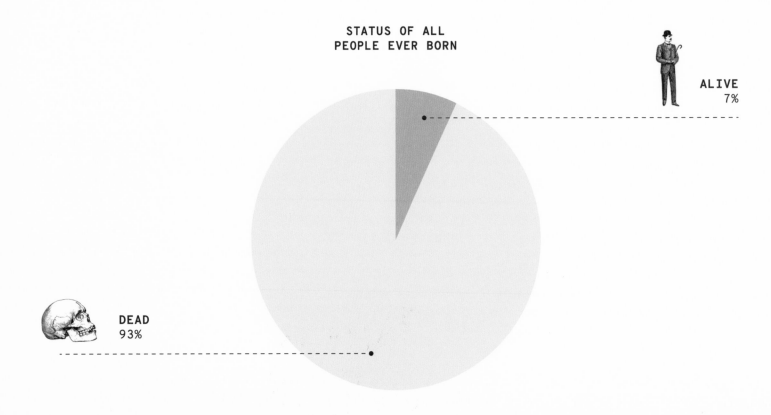

STATUS OF ALL
PEOPLE EVER BORN

ALIVE
7%

DEAD
93%

Source: "How Many People Have Lived on Earth?" Population Reference Bureau Washington, DC

3952 WEEKS (76 YEARS)

However, your time is finite—and a portion of it is already over.

RYAN GOSLING'S
POTENTIAL LIFE

● LIFE THAT IS OVER
○ LIFE THAT IS NOT OVER

Life is the sum total of our hours, days, months, and years between the dates "born" and "died." These are limited.

We don't control when our individual clock starts—or usually when it will end. However, you can make decisions about how you will use your limited time.

How finite?
Well, the odds of making it past 100 are slim.

Survival Rates (United States)　　　　　　　　　　　　　　　MEN　　WOMEN

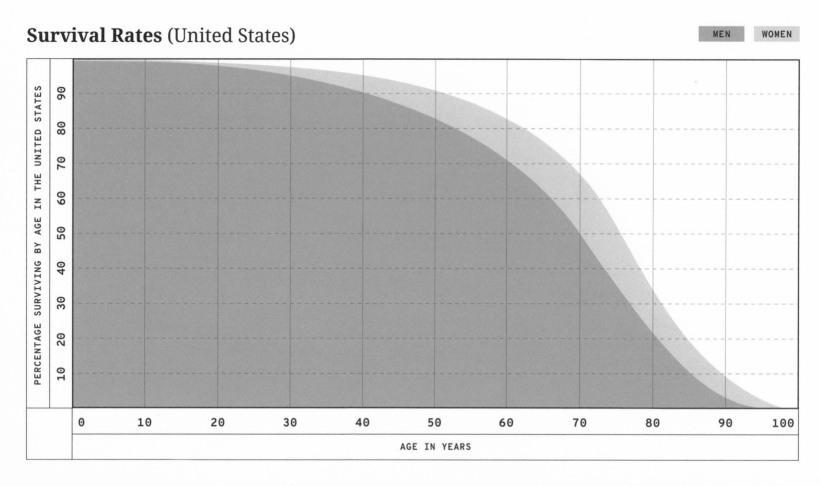

Source: "United States Life Tables 2017." CDC, National Vital Statistics Reports

So, how do we deal with this time constraint?

Some people simply ignore it and fail to act—or even act in counterproductive ways. Others stress over it, feeling anxious about something beyond their control. And although we'd like be to able to transcend this constraint, many of us just wing it: putting a little effort into thinking about it but mostly focusing on other things.

But if we truly embrace this time constraint, attempt to understand it, and plan for it, **we can achieve more with our lives.**

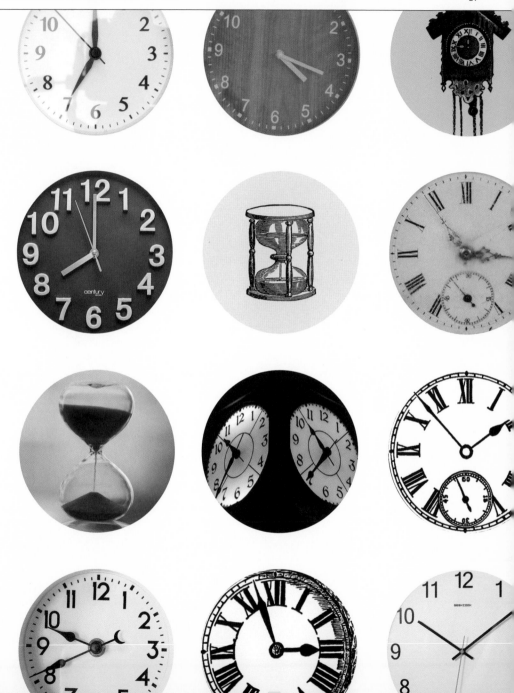

But what is it we're trying to achieve?

We all have different goals.

And many, many belief systems guide people in different ways.

Plus, most anything you can think of—and more that you can't.

BUDDHISM	Overcome suffering
CAPITALISM	Gain wealth
CHRISTIANITY	Love others—and Jesus—in order to reach heaven
CONSUMERISM	Seek stimulation and gain possessions
ENVIRONMENTALISM	Protect other species and the environment
EVOLUTION	Adapt to change and pass on your genetic code
NATIONALISM	Gain power
NIHILISM	Reject meaning
PREPPING	Survive and be resilient
SCIENCE	Understand reality
STOICISM	Find internal peace independent of external events

Most life goals are self-oriented and focused on the narrow window of time we're alive.

GOALS FOCUSED ON YOU IN YOUR LIFETIME

SEEK STIMULATION AND EXCITEMENT

GAIN WEALTH AND POSSESSIONS

PURSUE YOUR PASSIONS

EXPERIENCE NEW THINGS

EXPERIENCE SPECIFIC THINGS

BE CHALLENGED AND GROW

INCREASE SELF-AWARENESS AND ACCEPTANCE

ENJOY THE MOMENT

GAIN POWER

BELIEVE IN CERTAIN THINGS

SURVIVE AND BE RESILIENT

BE CONTENT AND AT PEACE

BE PRESENT IN THE MOMENT

UNDERSTAND REALITY

GAIN SOCIAL STATUS

. . .

A more holistic and impactful set of goals would call for you to look beyond yourself.

	GOALS FOCUSED ON YOU	GOALS FOCUSED ON OTHERS	GOALS FOCUSED ON THE WORLD
IN YOUR LIFETIME	PURSUE YOUR PASSIONS EXPERIENCE NEW THINGS BE CHALLENGED AND GROW . . .	LOVE OTHERS RAISE A HAPPY FAMILY INCREASE KNOWLEDGE . . .	CARE FOR OTHER LIFE FORMS STEWARD THE ENVIRONMENT PRACTICE MINDFUL CONSUMPTION . . .
BEYOND YOUR LIFETIME	REST EASY ETERNAL BLISS REINCARNATION (BUT OF COURSE, WHO REALLY KNOWS?)	ENSURE YOUR LEGACY (PASS ON KNOWLEDGE AND WEALTH) PASS ON YOUR GENES . . .	PRESERVE THE ENVIRONMENT FOR FUTURE GENERATIONS . . .

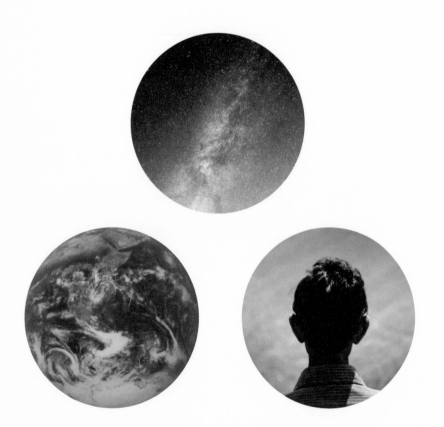

If we expand our goals in this way, we have the greatest opportunity to make our time here most impactful.

———

Finding balance among an expanded set of goals is a challenge that requires intentional thought and reflection—along with a solid understanding of who you are, what you value, and what you want to leave behind.

And the first step in spending our time well is to identfy and continually re-evaluate our goals.

Even when we have the most worthwhile goals, we encounter obstacles and roadblocks that get in our way. Let's understand the most common ones and figure out how to avoid them.

PART TWO

How can we avoid common problems in our lifetime?

Realizing That Life Ain't Easy

Life is full of problems, pitfalls, and setbacks.

We can't avoid them all.

———

We all hope to avoid the really big problems that could take us down or waste a lot of time. These include physical and mental health breakdowns, toxic relationships, excessive debt, and more.

Fortunately, there are strategies to make it through as unscathed as possible.

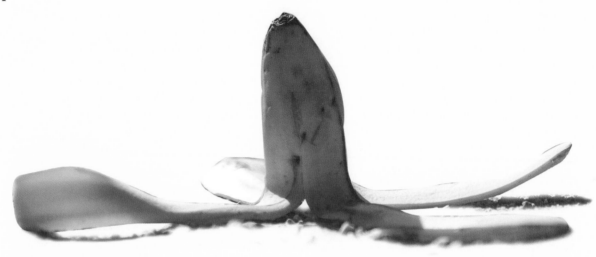

Think you got it tough?

You're not alone.
Encountering big problems is incredibly common.

1 Source: "About Chronic Diseases." CDC, National Center for Chronic Disease Prevention and Health Promotion
2 Source: "Key Facts: Obesity and Overweight." World Health Organization 2019
3 Source: "Study of Life Regrets." Remember a Charity
4 Source: "Mental Illness in the United States" National Institute of Mental Health
5 Source: "Marriage and divorce rates in the US." CDC, NCHS
6 Source: "Demographics and family status." 2017 United States Census
7 Source: Source: "Incarceration rates in America." FWD.us and Cornell University
8 Source: "Survey of loneliness." CIGNA 20208 http://www9.who.int/airpollution/en/
9 Source: "Piecing Together the Poverty Puzzle." World Bank 2019
10 Source: "Views on Race in America 2019." Pew Research
11 Source: "Ambient Air Pollution Database 2018." World Helath Organization
12 Source: "Has land use pushed terrestrial biodiversity beyond the planetary boundary? A global assessment." Journal of Science

WE EXPERIENCE PROBLEMS IN ALL PARTS OF LIFE

PHYSICAL
- 6 in 10 adults in the US have a chronic disease[1]
- 4 in 10 globally are overweight, with the percent of population who are obese trippling over the past 50 years[2]

MENTAL
- 4 in 10 regret their life choices[3]
- 1 in 5 US adults live with a mental illness. Roughly half remain untreated[4]

FAMILY
- 1 in 2 marriages end in divorce[5]
- 1 in 4 children live without a father in the home[6]
- 1 in 2 adults in America has had a family member in jail or prison[7]

FRIENDS
- 6 in 10 Americans report feeling lonely[8]

SOCIETY
- 1 in 2 people globally live on less than $6 a day and struggle to meet basic needs[9]
- 2 in 3 people say that it has become more common for people to express racist or racially insensitive views[10]

NATURAL RESOURCES
- 9 in 10 people globally live in places where air pollution exceeds World Health Organization guideline limits[11]

THE ENVIRONMENT
- Biodiversity on over half of the Earth's surface has dropped below a safe limit[12]

Our troubles stem from three main sources.
Most often, our troubles begin and end in our heads.

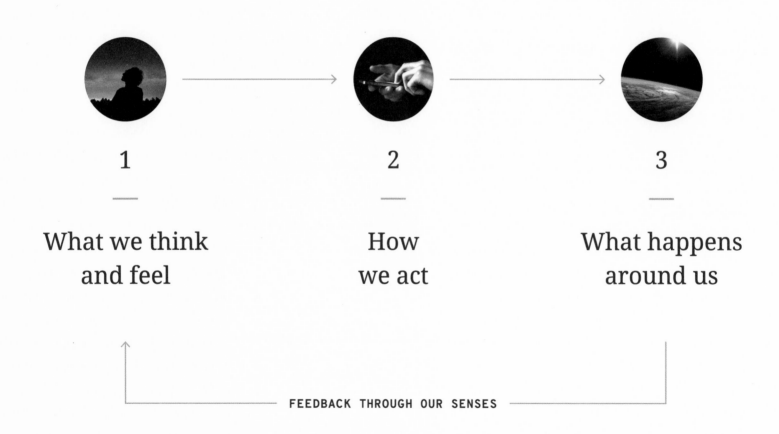

1	2	3
What we think and feel	How we act	What happens around us

FEEDBACK THROUGH OUR SENSES

Let's understand some common problems and identify how we can best deal with them.

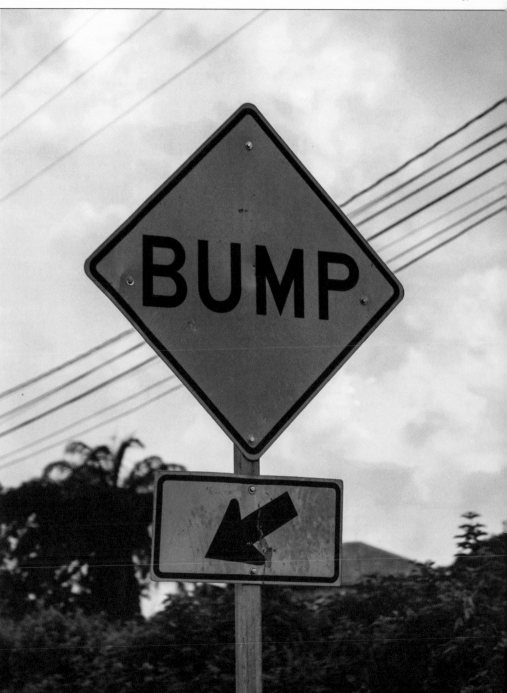

What we think and feel may misguide us...

SOURCE OF PROBLEM	EXAMPLES	WHY WE DO THIS	HOW TO DEAL WITH IT
Wrong Beliefs Many things that we believe may not be true; and we may, without questioning, take on belief systems others have created.	• Ideology • Superstitions • Many stories • Most things that can't be empirically observed or tested (e.g., ghosts)	Stories help us make sense of the world around us, feel more in control, and create social cohesion. When we're born, our brain is a fairly blank slate. To survive, we have to learn a lot quickly. It's more efficient to trust answers that others provide than to discover everything for ourselves.	Follow the scientific method (e.g., objectively test, measure, and validate theories). Be critical: ask ourselves, "Is it true?" Identify and consider counter-arguments. When we share our conclusions, ask for feedback.
Cognitive Bias Because our brains take shortcuts in processing information, we often make irrational and illogical decisions.	• Groupthink • Loss aversion • Anchoring • Over 150 additional documented ways in which we make errors in judgement	Our brains run on the equivalent of a few apples a day and need to conserve energy. As an energy-saving measure, we sometimes take shortcuts that deviate from logic.	Identify common cognitive biases, and check to see whether they play a part in our decision-making.
Misjudgement of Probabilities and Consequences We live in a complex system. We are pretty good at judging immediate consequences of actions but not second- or third-level consequences.	• Slippery slope of "just this once" ethical lapses • Butterfly effect of cascading consequences	Our understanding of cause and effect relationships is often limited by our lack of experience or the complexity of factors involved.	Recognize that things might not work as planned. Identify any extreme risks. Consider the likely causes and consequences of our own actions and the actions of those around us.

...and may leave us **feeling unfulfilled**.

SOURCE OF PROBLEM	EXAMPLES	WHY WE DO THIS	HOW TO DEAL WITH IT
Adaptation Changes in our situation do not necessarily lead to long-term sustainable happiness.	• Getting a raise • Buying things (new house, clothes, toys)	We mistakenly believe that more possessions will lead to sustained happiness.	**Focus on inner happiness vs. externally driven stimulation.** **Prioritize experiences over things.**
Ignorance There's a lot that we know we don't know (i.e., the unknown)—and far more that we may not be aware that we don't know (i.e., the *unknown* unknowns).	• Future events • Things outside of our area of competence	We haven't invested the necessary time or mental energy (because we won't or can't).	**Be selective about and invest in the areas we need to become insightful in.** **Recognize that there's a lot we don't know.**
Conflicting Values & Priorities We have multiple values that often conflict with each other. Even when we prioritize effectively, these conflicting values create angst.	• Authentic feedback vs. ego-building praise • Work vs. family • Self vs. others • Self vs. planet	We can't have it all due to constraints (primarily time). Our brain has developed to be good at some taks (e.g., keeping us alive) but not at others (e.g., quickly and accurately calculating complex probabilities).	**Determine what's most important to you.** **Find ways to reconcile conflicting values.** **Accept that we may need to make trade-offs—but make them wisely.**
External vs. Internal Validation Because we often look to others to give us affirmation and sense of worth, we often don't act in ways that are true to ourselves.	• Comparing ourselves to others • Needing praise in order for us to be happy • Making happiness conditional on external events	Throughout most of human history, our ancestors who lost status or were evicted from their tribe faced consequences that were often fatal.	**Limit exposure to social media.** **Build self-confidence and a sense of self-worth.** **Cultivate meaningful relationships.**

How we act may prevent us from achieving our most important goals.

SOURCE OF PROBLEM	EXAMPLES	WHY WE DO THIS	HOW TO DEAL WITH IT
Instant Gratification Some things that cause us to feel good in the moment may cause problems for us or others in the future. Because we usually want more of what initially brings us pleasure, we have a tough time defining and stoping at "enough."	• Binge drinking • Substance abuse • Junk food • Gambling • Checking our phone • Getting "likes" on social media	Our brain rewards certain survival-oriented behavior with dopamine hits. Our brain reward system hasn't fully adapted to the modern world, where hard-to-get things (e.g., sugar) are plentiful and always available. We fall into a loop of overindulging to the point of harming ourselves.	**Avoid temptation (e.g., don't have junk food around the house).** **Reflect on our longer-term goals.** **Practice moderation.**
Laziness We may not always do the things that we know we should do.	• Procrastination • Failure to show up or get started	As a survival mechanism, we are hard-wired to conserve energy for the most critical needs because food (i.e., energy) could be scarce.	**Use to-do lists.** **Have an accountability partner.** **Set goal reminders.** **Get started, develop a plan, break big things into a series of small tasks, and tackle them one by one.** **Focus on overall well-being (e.g., sleep, diet, exercise).**
Weakness We may not always have the ability or strength to achieve what we want.	• Failure to reach a workout goal • Difficulty building rewarding relationships	No one is born great at everything. We become stronger by being challenged, failing, and growing.	**Continue to challenge ourselves and grow.** **Seek support from others whose distinct talents can offset our weaknesses.**

What **happens around us** may be beyond our control—but not our influence.

SOURCE OF PROBLEM	EXAMPLES	WHY THIS HAPPENS	HOW TO DEAL WITH IT
Bad Luck Events happen outside of our control.	• Rain on a wedding day • Car accident	The world is imperfect. The only way to eliminate risk is to live in a hermetically sealed room. The more we do and the longer we live, the more likely it is that some negative things will happen beyond our control.	Don't put ourselves in situations where bad luck could be catastrophic (e.g., sailing in bad weather).
Others Don't Treat Us as We Feel We Deserve to Be Treated People don't always do what we'd like them to do.	• Someone is unkind or takes advantage of us	We influence—but don't control—the behavior of others. People have complex motivations—and the same flaws we do.	Avoid toxic relationships. Recognize that others are struggling with their own problems. Reciprocity works: treat others well.
The Complexity of the World Surprises Us The world is an extremely interconnected and complex system.	• Black swan events (i.e., something beyond what is normally expected with potentially severe consequences) • Unanticipated second- or third-level consequences	Many things are random and beyond our control.	Think beyond primary consequences. Think about the probability of each potential outcome. Recognize that low-probability events still happen.

PART THREE

How can we make the most of our time?

Improving Our Quality, Quantity, and Perception of Time

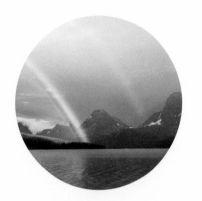

Increase Quality

———

Allocate our time well, and get the greatest benefit for the time spent.

There are three ways to make the most of our time in life.

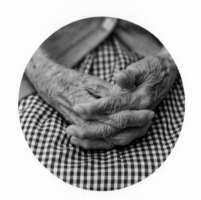

Maximize Quantity

———

Stay healthy—and avoid an early death.

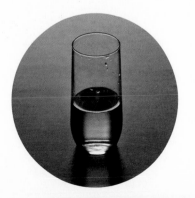

Enhance Perception

———

Learn to slow down, speed up, and savor time.

Increase Quality

Although each day only has 24 hours and each week has only 7 days, we can achieve the greatest return on our limited time in two main ways:

1. By allocating time wisely
Invest more time in higher-value areas. Spend more time in areas that provide enjoyment in the moment, as well as longer-term benefit to ourselves and others. (Spend less time in areas that don't make us happy.)

2. By using time efficiently
Make the most of our time by figuring out what works and what doesn't in any given area (e.g., work, sleep, leisure). Then put that knowledge into practice.

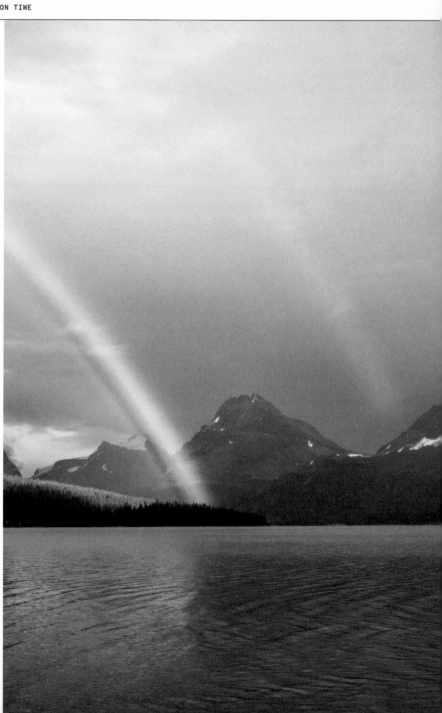

Let's start with how we allocate our time.

Doing it well is like juggling.

—

When you balance everything effectively, it feels and looks effortless. But finding this sense of flow doesn't just happen. If you don't pay attention, you may drop the ball (literally and figuratively).

Although you can only do one or two things at a time, you have to think about what's happening with everything else. At a certain point, the more you take on, the harder it becomes to keep everything going.

To juggle successfully and to allocate our time well, we need to practice, try new things, give ourselves permission to fail, and refine our technique based on what we discover works and what doesn't.

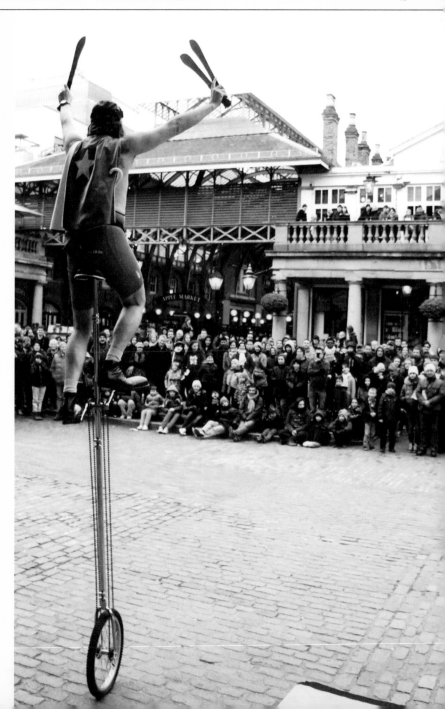

When we zoom out, life seems like a blank canvas that we can fill up any way that we want.

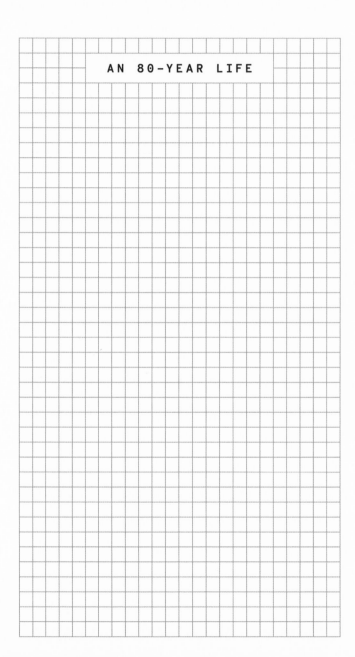

AN 80-YEAR LIFE

☐ = ONE MONTH

☐ = ONE MONTH

AN 80-YEAR LIFE

SLEEP (~33%)

WORK (~13%)

SCHOOL (~3%)

COMMUTE/CHORES(~8%)

LEISURE TIME (~42%)

Well, not exactly.

A lot of the time in your life has been—or will be—decided for you.

The rest of your life goes here: time with friends, with family, and by yourself.

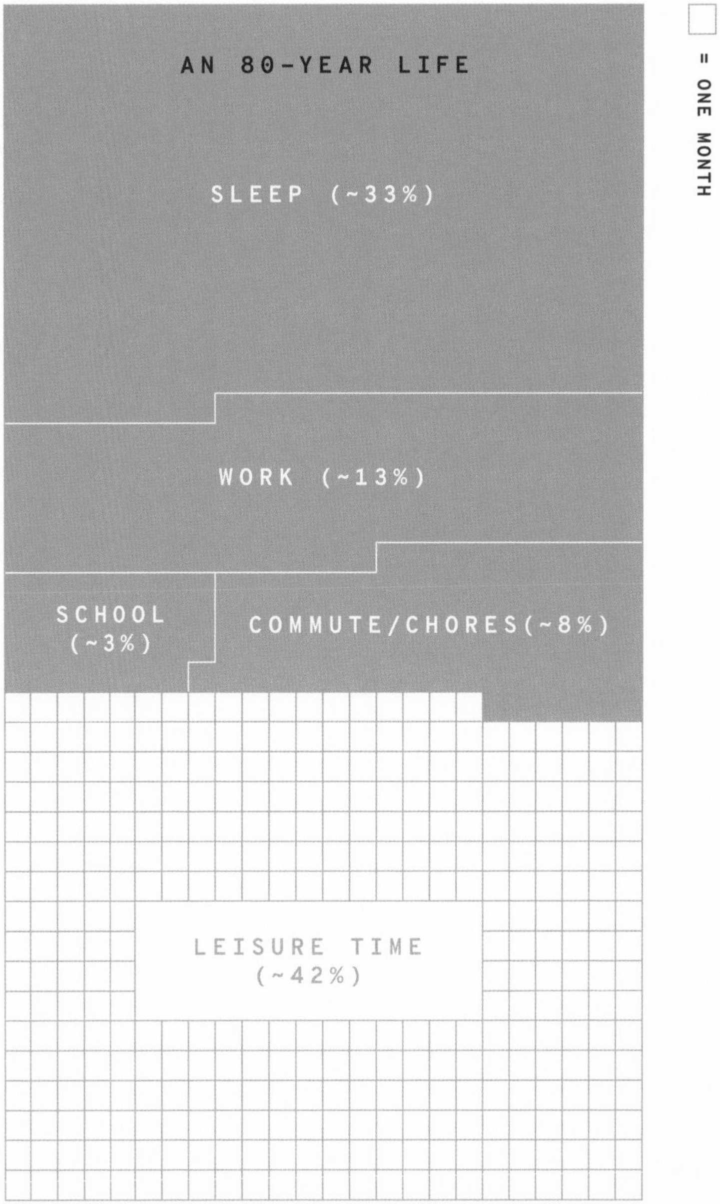

That leisure time is highly valuable.

Historically, leisure time was for living life to the fullest through intellectual or creative pursuits.

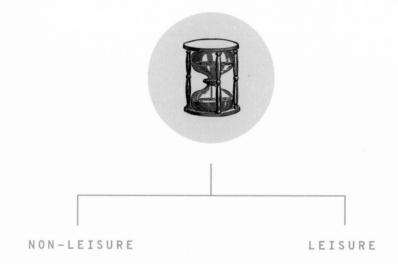

NON—LEISURE

Self-Oriented Time

Work, politics, and other activities to advance your own interests.

LEISURE

Truth-Oriented Time

Pursuit of truth, goodness, and beauty in the world and in one another.

✳ *The Greek word for leisure, scholé, meant "a place for learning."*

HOW TIME IS
CONCEPTUALIZED NOW

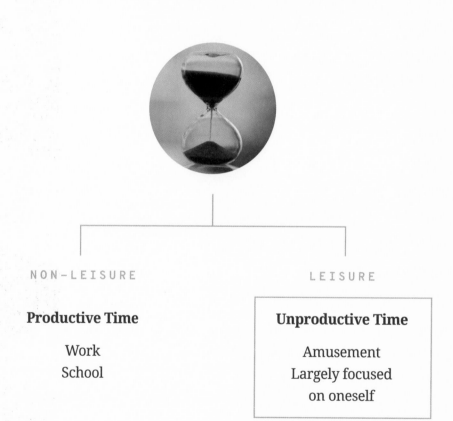

Nowadays, most of
us think of leisure as
lounging around and
doing nothing.

NON-LEISURE

Productive Time

Work
School

LEISURE

Unproductive Time

Amusement
Largely focused
on oneself

For centuries, our ancestors engaged in a variety of leisure activities that we now know contribute to well-being.

- Family gatherings

- Growing and preparing food

- Outdoor recreation

- Sports and physical activity

- Faith

- Reading

- Hobbies

- Socializing

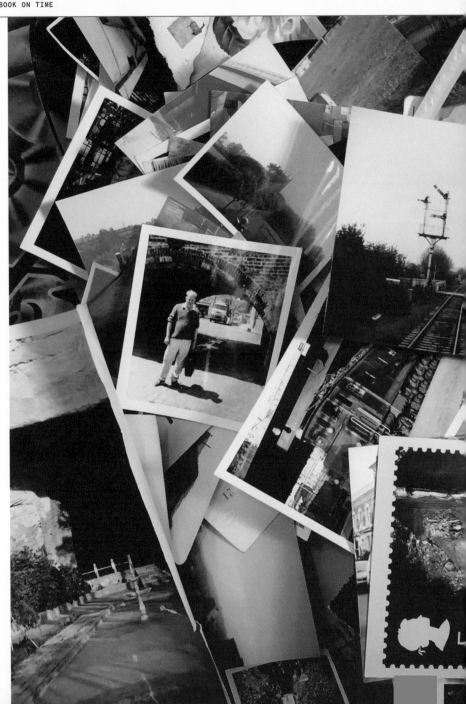

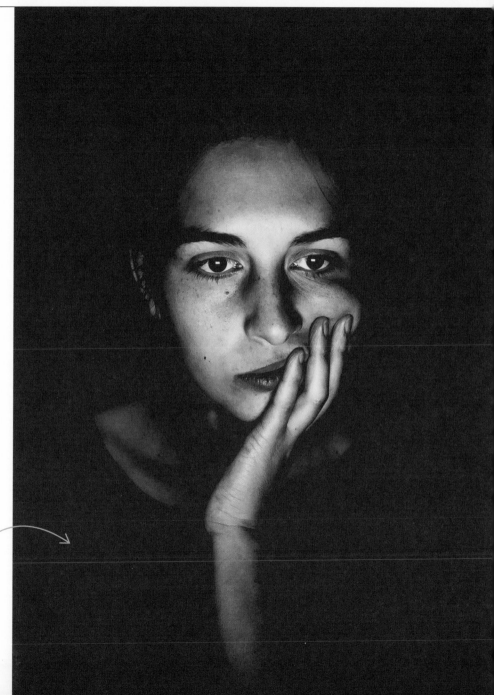

But technology has led us to re-allocate a lot of that time.

Our leisure time has now mostly become screen time.

We spend up to 9 hours a day (including most of our leisure time) staring at screens.

Source: "United States Life Tables 2017." CDC, National Vital Statistics Reports

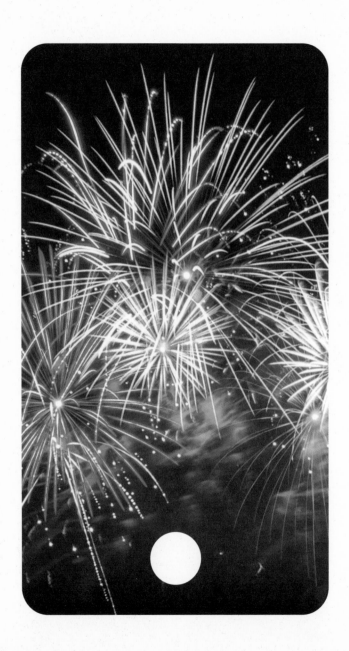

That's not to say it's all bad.

We get some amazing benefits
from screen time.

———

Screen time can provide information, entertainment,
connection, convenience, and more.

It also stimulates sight, our dominant sense
for processing external information.

But there's a problem.
It's designed to be addictive.

A small but mounting body of evidence demonstrates that smartphones and other forms of screen time are addictive.

Research also suggests that screen time may actually be rewiring physical aspects of our brain.

When people are separated from their phone for a single day, they often report anxiety and withdrawal-type symptoms.

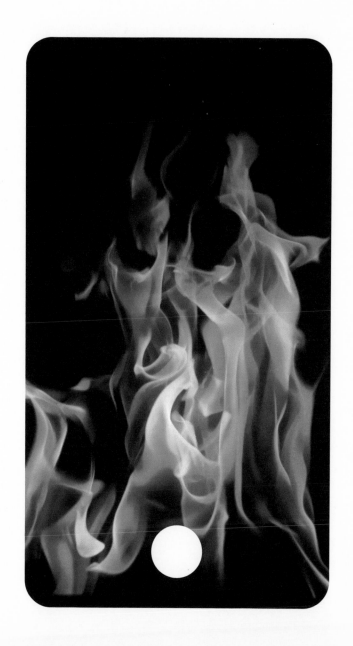

Source: "Screen time and the Brain." Harvard Medical School, Center on Media and Child Health at Boston Children's Hospital; "Irresistible: The Rise of Addictive Technology and the Business of Keeping Us Hooked" Dr. Adam Alter NYU

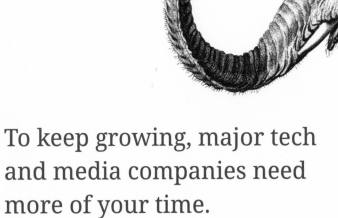

To keep growing, major tech and media companies need more of your time.

And they're poised to take it from you.

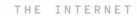

LITTLE OLD YOU

Trying to stay connected while protecting your leisure time.

THE INTERNET

Fueled by Big Tech. Thousands of specialists building products powered by advanced machine learning, big data, and A/B testing to get more of your time and "engagement."

And your most valuable asset (your leisure time and attention) is being sold to advertisers.

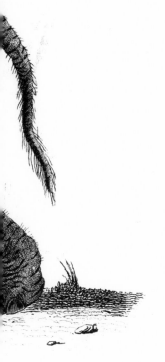

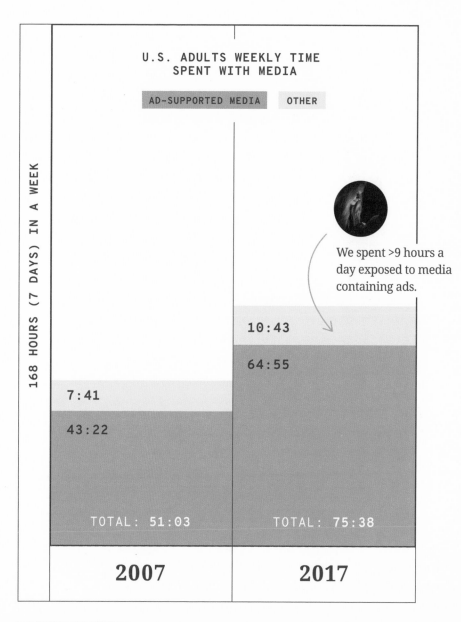

U.S. ADULTS WEEKLY TIME SPENT WITH MEDIA

AD-SUPPORTED MEDIA   OTHER

168 HOURS (7 DAYS) IN A WEEK

We spent >9 hours a day exposed to media containing ads.

2007
7:41
43:22
TOTAL: 51:03

2017
10:43
64:55
TOTAL: 75:38

Source: "Total Audience Report 2018." Nielson

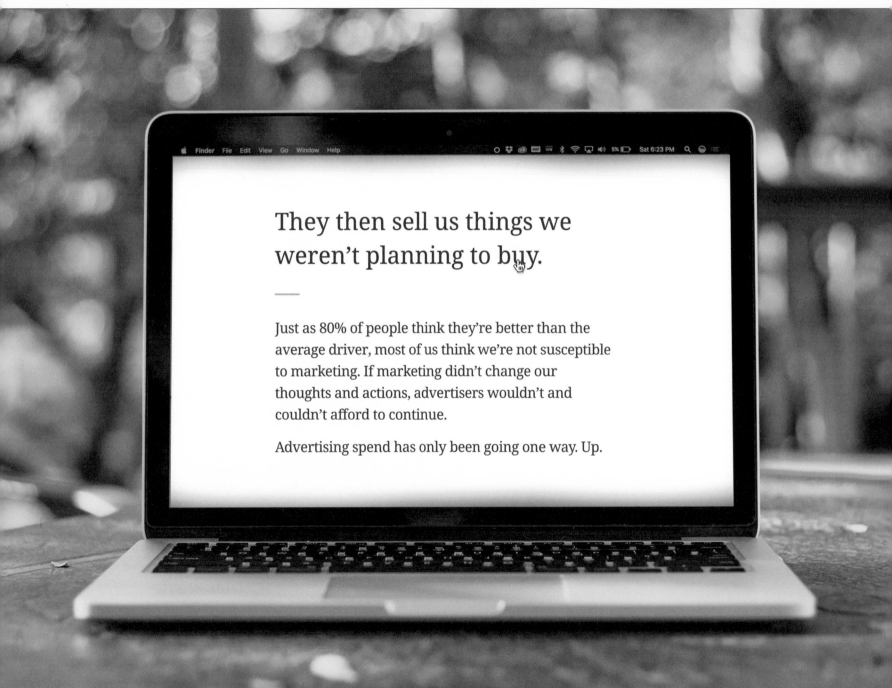

They then sell us things we weren't planning to buy.

———

Just as 80% of people think they're better than the average driver, most of us think we're not susceptible to marketing. If marketing didn't change our thoughts and actions, advertisers wouldn't and couldn't afford to continue.

Advertising spend has only been going one way. Up.

Which creates a cycle that sacrifices our leisure time.

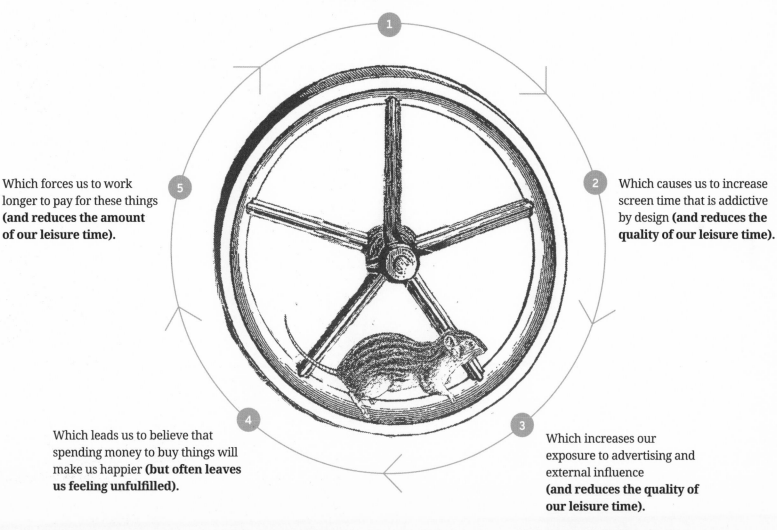

1 — We try to escape stress with quick and easy distractions.

2 — Which causes us to increase screen time that is addictive by design **(and reduces the quality of our leisure time).**

3 — Which increases our exposure to advertising and external influence **(and reduces the quality of our leisure time).**

4 — Which leads us to believe that spending money to buy things will make us happier **(but often leaves us feeling unfulfilled).**

5 — Which forces us to work longer to pay for these things **(and reduces the amount of our leisure time).**

And if time is money, then money is an exchange for and claim on our time—and other people's time.

In practice, money serves as a means of exchange for goods and services that we can use now or in the future.

The primary input to both goods and services is people's time. When we pay for something, we're mostly compensating someone for the time it took them to find raw materials, gather them, and produce goods or provide services.

But remember: money can never give you back the time you spent trying to get it.

We can use money (i.e., purchase other people's time) in order to improve the quality of our own time.

Use money to:

- Reallocate your time
  (e.g., do less housekeeping)

- Make the most of your time
  (e.g., get a massage on vacation)

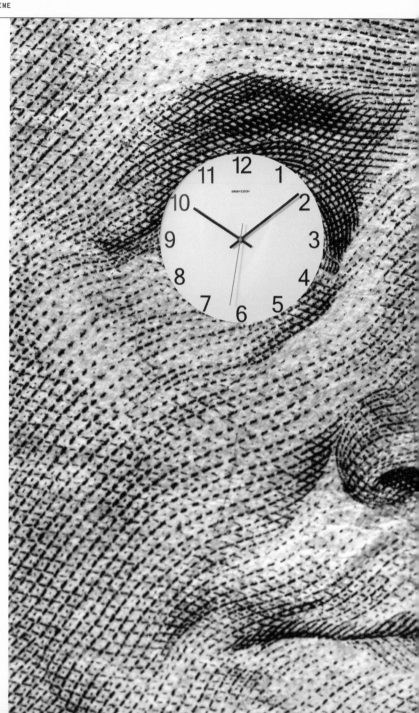

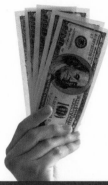

There are five ways to get money. (We recommend the clean and capitalist ways).

	HOW WE GET MONEY	EXAMPLES	WHAT IT REQUIRES
The "Clean" Way	Provide a product or service that people willingly pay us for because they need or want it.	• Frontline workers • Salaried employees • Entrepreneurs	• Creating something of value to others • Mutual agreement on price
The "Capitalist" Way	Give people money now in exchange for getting more back later.	• Investors • Rent seekers	• Capital to start with • People who want and can repay your money
The "Lucky" Way	Receive money because of who we are or something we gambled on.	• Trust-fund kids • Inheritance recipients • Lottery winners • Speculators	• Circumstances largely outside of your control
The "Dirty" Way	Take it from people against their will using theft, deception, and/or violence.	• Thieves • Counterfeiters • Fraudsters	• Victims • Ability to get away with it
The "I'm King" Way	Require that people give us money or else they will be punished (e.g., fined, imprisoned, killed). May provide services in return.	• Mob bosses • Dictators • The taxman	• Ability to set and enforce the rules

When you're ready to re-allocate some of that screen time, **don't forget to get away.**

———

Maybe we're biased, since this is our jam after all, but truly, a simple break from the day-to-day is one of the most beneficial ways to re-allocate your time. It's a lot easier to recharge and reconnect when you're out of your normal environment and routine.

Find somewhere that provides the space and time that you need to relax. We think that the best getaways provide experiences that are good for the mind and body.

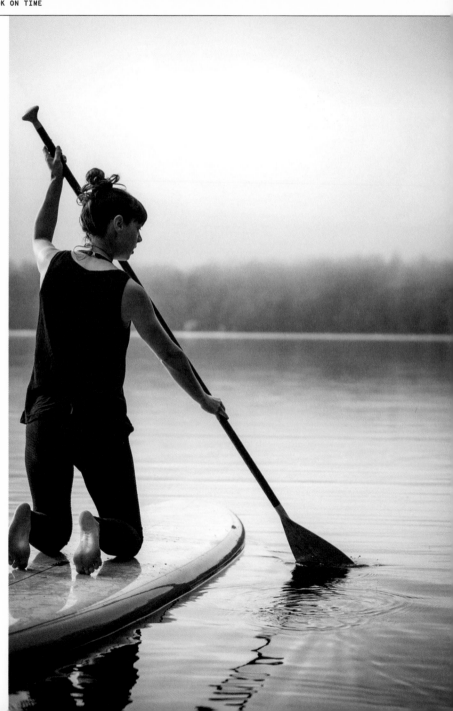

To summarize, here's how we recommend improving your **time allocation.**

Understand where your time goes. The first step is becoming aware of how you spend your time. Reflect on the past few days, weeks, and months.

Reflect on what you really do and don't want in life. Take the time to think about your values and goals—and whether or not you're on track. You can have most anything you want—but you can't have everything.

Evaluate different options for spending your time. Understand the options, and determine which are more or less likely to help you get what you want.

Develop and implement a plan. (Keep it simple.) We recommend listing the things you will stop, start, and continue. Don't overlook the power of doing less.

Trade money for time. Although money comes and goes, time isn't replaceable. Consider outsourcing your lower-value, time-consuming activities.

Recognize flow and interdependencies. Getting time allocation right feels like juggling well without dropping critical things. Also, spending time in some areas impacts others. For example, more exercise often cascades to better sleep, diet, and mental well-being.

Schedule a getaway. Life gets crazy sometimes—and goes by fast. Maintain regularly scheduled breaks where you get away from it all to recalibrate. We recommend that you go somewhere relaxing and inspiring at least once every three months.

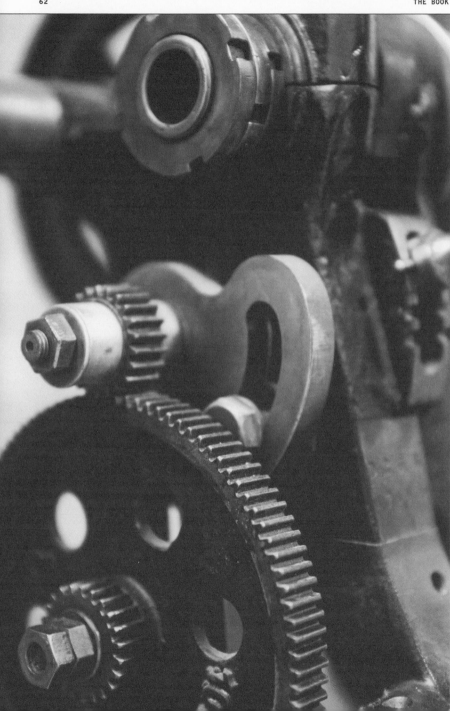

Which brings us to
efficiency.

If you're going to spend
time on something, do it
well so that you get the
most benefit.

—

By making a few scientifically supported changes,
you can capture more benefit from the areas in
which you invest time.

ABOUT 90% OF OUR
TIME GOES HERE

Where does the time go?

———

Well, for the most part it goes into these common categories. So, let's dive deep into each one and learn how to benefit the most from each.

Sleeping

Eating

Exercise

Education & Work

Leisure & Vacation

Romance & Family

Sleeping

If you think **sleeping** is a waste of time, think again.

During our lifetime, we spend roughly 234,000 hours sleeping. Our bodies are quite busy while we snooze the night away.

When we sleep, memory consolidates and solidifies, growth hormones are secreted, toxins are cleared from the brain, and emotions fade away and become more stable.

During this crucial time, our bodies also work to restore themselves, including valuable muscle repair. And regular sleep patterns exert a strong influence on healthy immune functions.

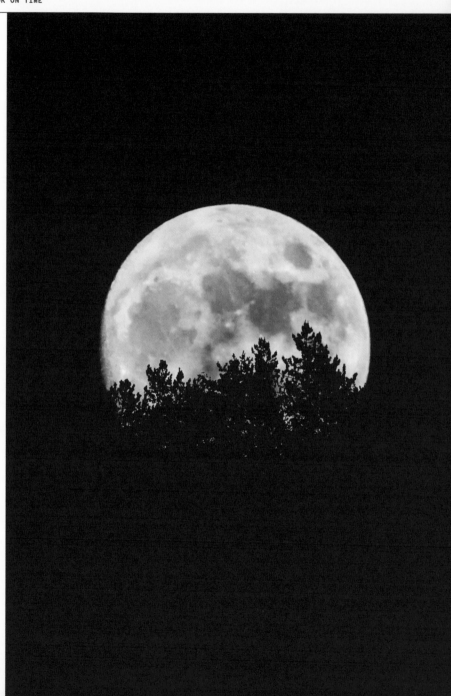

In fact, sleep is so important that **sleep deprivation** is a form of torture whether you do it to yourself or are captured by hostile enemy forces.

EFFECTS OF SLEEP DEPRIVATION

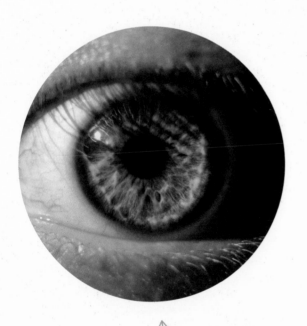

Short-Term Impact

- Impaired cognitive performance and memory
- Loss of concentration and productivity
- Increased appetite
- Decreased ability to handle social situations
- Loss of emotional control

Long-Term Impact

- Decline in memory
- High propensity for weight gain and diabetes
- Mood swings, depression, and mental illness
- Weakened immune system
- Higher propensity for inflammation
- Greater risk of cardiovascular diseases
- Potentially, premature death

Even moderate lack of sleep can cause cognitive and physical impairment at levels similar to being drunk.

Sources: "Sleep Deprivation and Deficiency." NIH National Lung, Heart, and Blood Institute, "Moderate sleep deprivation produces impairments equivalent to alcohol intoxication" A M Williamson, Anne-Marie Feyer

Don't deprive yourself.
More sleep would do a lot of people good.

—

Many of us don't sleep enough.

- Over the last 30 years, the average sleep duration around the world has decreased.

- More than 1 in 3 US adults short-change their sleep on a regular basis.

- 7 in 10 high school students get fewer than the recommended 8 hours of sleep.

- 1 in 3 Americans suffer from sleep disorders.

- 1 in 3 Americans admit to having fallen asleep behind the wheel.

- Car crashes due to untreated cases of Obstructive Sleep Apnea (OSA) cost nearly $16 billion.

Sources: "Sleep Deprivation and Deficiency." NIH National Lung, Heart, and Blood Institute, "Moderate sleep deprivation produces impairments equivalent to alcohol intoxication" A M Williamson, Anne-Marie Feyer, "Behavioral Risk Factor Surveillance System" CDC, The American Academy of Sleep Medicine, the Sleep Research Society, "Sleep Disorders as a Cause of Motor Vehicle Collisions." International Journal of Preventative Medicine

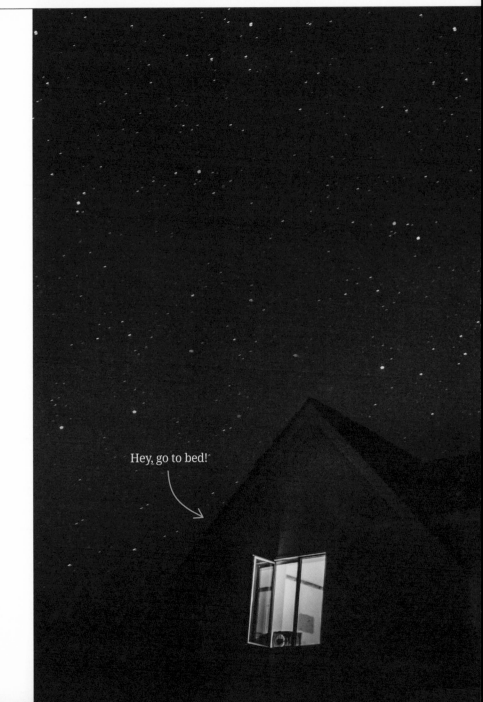

Hey, go to bed!

How much sleep should you get?

AGE	RECOMMENDED	NOT RECOMMENDED
0-3 months old	14 to 17 hours	Less than 11 hours More than 19 hours
4-11 months old	12 to 15 hours	Less than 10 hours More than 18 hours
1-2 years old	11 to 14 hours	Less than 9 hours More than 16 hours
3-5 years old	10 to 13 hours	Less than 8 hours More than 14 hours
6-13 years old	9 to 11 hours	Less than 7 hours More than 12 hours
14-17 years old	8 to 10 hours	Less than 7 hours More than 11 hours
18-25 years old	7 to 9 hours	Less than 6 hours More than 11 hours
26-64 years old	7 to 9 hours	Less than 6 hours More than 10 hours
65+ years old	7 to 8 hours	Less than 5 hours More than 9 hours

Source: "Are You Getting Enough Sleep?" CDC

And of course, quantity isn't always quality.

—

How to tell if you don't have healthy sleep habits:

- Taking more than 30 minutes to fall asleep

- Regularly waking up multiple times during the night

- Waking up for more than 20 minutes during the night

- Trouble waking up on time without an alarm clock

- Experiencing extreme daytime drowsiness

- Falling asleep at the wheel or on commutes

- Consistently taking naps longer than an hour

Source: "How to Determine if You Need Better Sleep." SleepFoundation.org

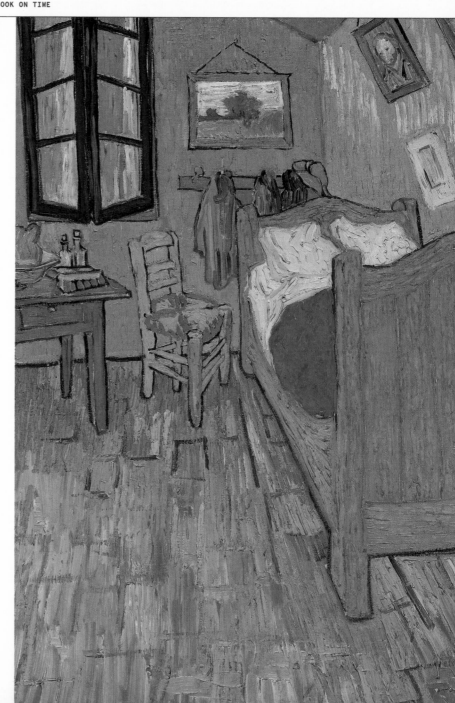

What else can prevent good sleep?

—

Many factors contribute to poor quality sleep.
A few to be aware of:

Electronics placed close by the bed
They can emit light or vibrations that affect quality
of sleep and disrupt your circadian rhythm. Also,
the closer your phone is to the bed, the greater the
temptation to check it.

Discomfort
If you consistently experience joint pain after
waking up, your mattress and/or sleep position
may be ready for a change.

Undetected or untreated sleep disorders
Medical conditions like Obstructive Sleep Apnea
(OSA) or Chronic Insomnia are very disruptive to
quality sleep.

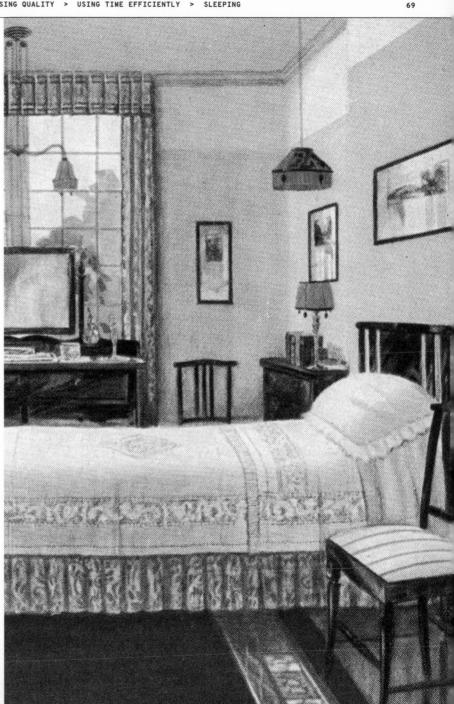

Setting yourself up for a **successful night's sleep.**

AREAS TO IMPROVE	HOW TO DO IT
Your Schedule By keeping your bedtime routine consistent, you can help maintain your circadian rhythm.	• Generally, find a bedtime between 8PM and midnight. • Take 10-30 minute naps in the early afternoon (3-5PM), which can help increase alertness and emotional control. • Longer naps are also helpful but may increase periods of grogginess after you wake up. • Beware of excessive daytime napping, which may be a signal of health concerns.
Your Environment For blissful sleep, optimize your den in pursuit of zen.	• Keep your sleeping environment as noise-free as possible. • Listen to white noise, ocean sounds, or soothing music. • Avoid sources of light, especially blue light emitted by electronics. • Increase exposure to bright light in the morning—this can improve subsequent sleep quality. • Keep humidity in the 40-60% range, consistent with daytime comfort levels. • Adjust room temperature to 60-67 degrees Fahrenheit (15-20 Celsius) or slightly warmer. • Maintain thermo-neutrality by adjusting ambient temperature and adding layers of insulating materials. • Ensure your bedroom is well ventilated with plenty of oxygen. • Try inhaling essential oils, especially lavender, to improve sleep quality.
Your Ritual A good bedtime ritual can help you fall asleep easier.	• Avoid electronics for an hour before going to bed. • Avoid eating or drinking (alcohol and other fluids) right before bed. • Allow yourself to exercise before bed. It may increase body temperature but shows no effect on sleep. • Wind down by reading (not electronic), massage, mindfulness exercises, or meditation. • Relax with a bath, shower, or even dipping feet in warm water.

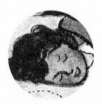

Still need a little extra help?

Gear up for better sleep with scientifically supported goods.

Weighted blankets can improve sleep quality for insomniacs and those who may be autistic.

Ear plugs and **eye masks** reduce visual and audio disturbances during sleep.

Socks or footed pajamas can improve sleep quality by keeping your feet warm.

Melatonin supplements may be effective, especially if you have jet-lag or insomnia.

Different **mattresses** may be optimal for different people. Firmer mattresses may be better if you're experiencing back pain.

Ginkgo biloba supplements may improve sleep for people suffering from depression. **Glycine**, the amino acid, may improve sleep quality.

Autonomous Sensory Meridian Response (ASMR) videos help some people fall asleep quickly.

Ergonomic pillows & blankets may help, although academic research is scarce. But hey—whatever gets your snooze on! Different **sleep positions** may be optimal for different people. Lying on your back (supine) may be best for your joints but harmful for sleep apnea. Sleeping on your side (lateral) may be best for clearing toxins from the brain.

Source: Cleveland Clinic, NIH, Harvard Medical School, Mayo Clinic

Eating

How can we make the most out of our time **eating?**

During our lifetime, we spend roughly 35,040 hours eating. Whole days, holidays, vacations, meetings, dates, and countless other activities center around meals.

They can be communal or individual, pleasurable or stressful. Either way, we need to eat—and we spend a lot of time thinking about, preparing, and eating our meals.

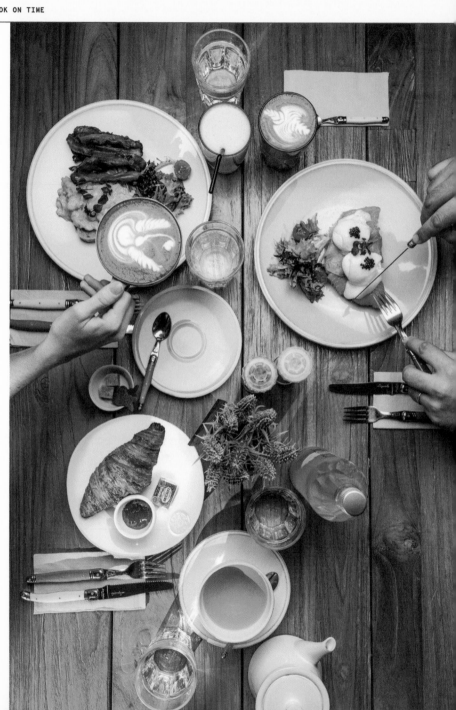

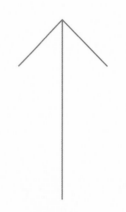

EATING WELL
INCREASES

Overall health
Cognition
Digestive health
Sleep

"An apple a day keeps the doctor away."

It's true. What you put in your body has a big impact on the quality and length of your life.

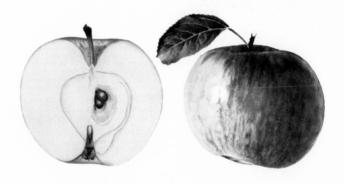

EATING WELL
DECREASES CHANCES OF

Cancer
Diabetes
Heart attacks and strokes
Obesity

Source: "The benefits of good nutrition." U.S. Department of Health and Human Services

What does **eating well** mean?

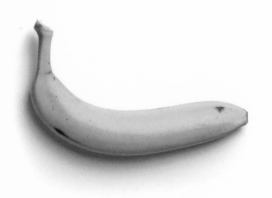

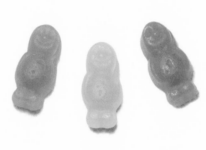

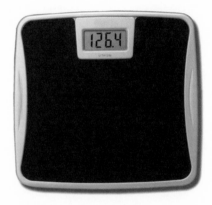

Eat More Real Food

—

Eat mostly unprocessed whole foods like whole grains, fruits, and vegetables. The natural fibers in these foods decrease hunger, slow digestion, and feed good digestive bacteria.

Eat Less Fake Food

—

Although it takes a lot of self-control, try to reduce fructose from processed desserts, sugary drinks, and alcohol. (Because the liver can't process excess fructose well, it contributes to diabetes and fatty-liver disease).

Additionally, decrease salt (which is necessary for your nervous system but can cause hypertension and kidney damage) and decrease saturated fat from red meat.

Ditch the Fad Diets

—

Studies of overweight/obese people who were put on diets high in fat and low in carbs, or vice versa, revealed similar weight-loss results. The key is to eat a balanced diet and to not overeat.

We used to know what we put in our bodies because we grew our food.

American Workforce in Agriculture

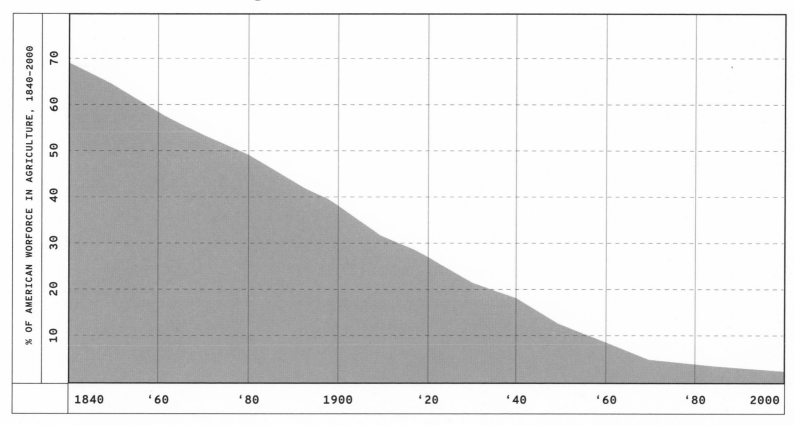

Source: "Work: Employment & Labor Force Participation." USDA.

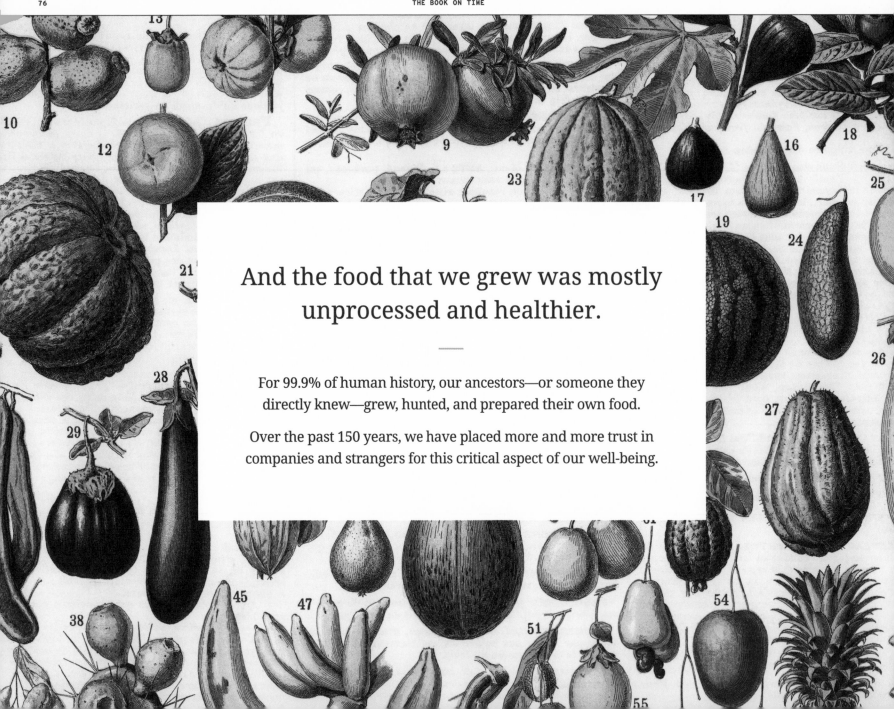

And the food that we grew was mostly unprocessed and healthier.

———

For 99.9% of human history, our ancestors—or someone they directly knew—grew, hunted, and prepared their own food.

Over the past 150 years, we have placed more and more trust in companies and strangers for this critical aspect of our well-being.

As big conglomerates started manufacturing our food, they loaded it up with sugar and sweeteners.

Added Sweetener Consumption (pounds per person)

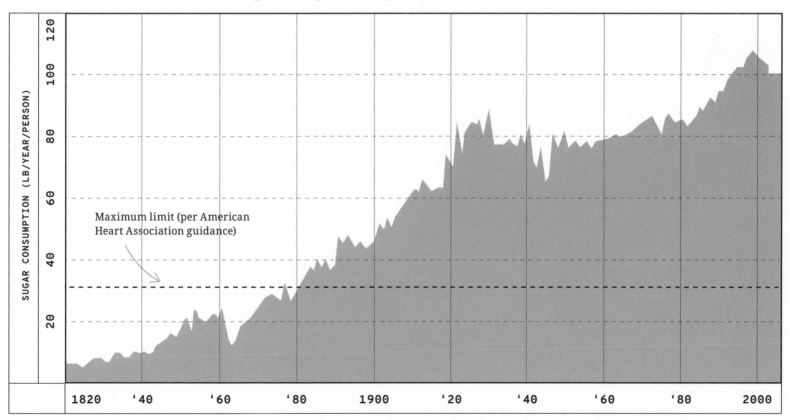

Sources: "Added Sugar Guidelines." The American Heart Association, Sugar consumption in the US diet." Stephan Guyenet, Jeremy Landen

Select corporate revenues (in billions)

	1985	2000	2010
Coca-Cola	8B	21B	**35B**
pepsi	~8B	20B	**58B**
McDonald's	4B	14B	**16B**
General Mills	4B	5B	**15B**

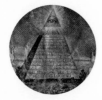

Corporate revenues
became fat.

Source: Corporate annual reports

And so did most
of America.

Obesity rates in the United States

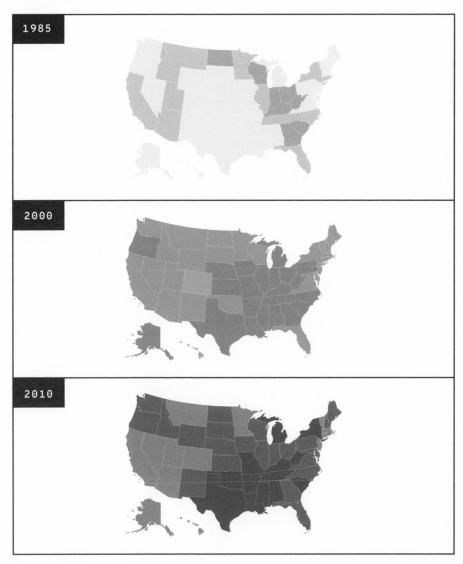

NO DATA
<10%
10%–14%
15%–19%
20%–24%
25%–29%
≥30%

Source: "Adult Obesity Prevalence Maps." CDC

Sugar sure is addictive. In lab experiments, 94% of rats choose sugar over cocaine.

———

Numerous studies have linked sugar and processed foods
to a range of nasty outcomes:

Short-term:

- Reduced energy and focus
- Sugar crash including headaches and nausea
- Indigestion and acid reflux
- Poor sleep

Long-term:

- Obesity and diabetes
- Depression
- Digestive issues
- Teeth and bone issues
- Heart disease and stroke
- Cancer
- Early death

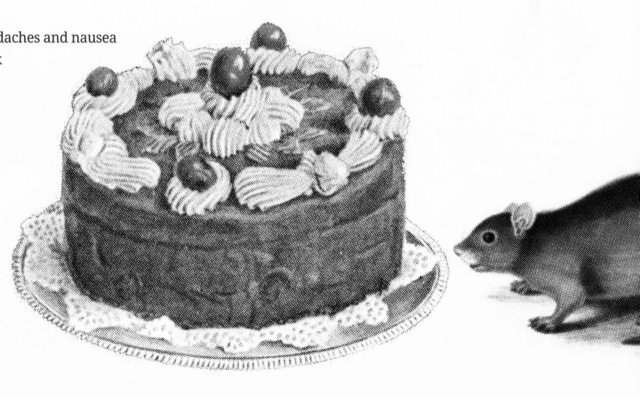

Source: "Intense sweetness surpasses cocaine reward." Lenoir M, Serre F, Cantin L, Ahmed SH (2007)

Sugar is **even worse** in liquid form.

Drink water, not calorie filled beverages.

———

Because the brain doesn't register liquids as it does solid foods, we frequently overconsume beverages.

In one study, participants who replaced a solid meal with a liquid one that contained the same number of calories consumed 10-20% more calories over the next 24 hours.

6 APPLES HAVE THE SAME NUMBER OF CALORIES
AS AN 8-OUNCE CUP OF APPLE JUICE

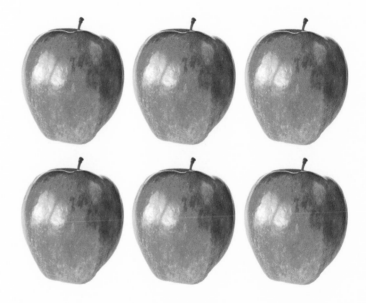

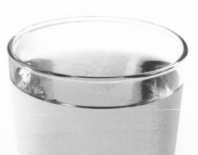

Sources: "Neurobiology of circadian rhythm regulation." Alan Rosenwasser, Fred Turek, "Solid versus liquid calories: current scientific understandings." Janice Lee, Richard Mattes

And watch the snack attack.

More and more snacks seem to be finding their way into our diets. Snack-time foods have more calories per gram than our meal-time foods.

Often, snacking is induced by cravings that we find hard to control. You can fight these cravings by keeping on hand healthier snack foods, being mindful of what you're snacking on, and limiting frequency of snacking.

Source: "Hypercaloric diets with increased meal frequency, but not meal size, increase intrahepatic triglycerides."
Koopman KE, Caan MW, Nederveen AJ, et al.

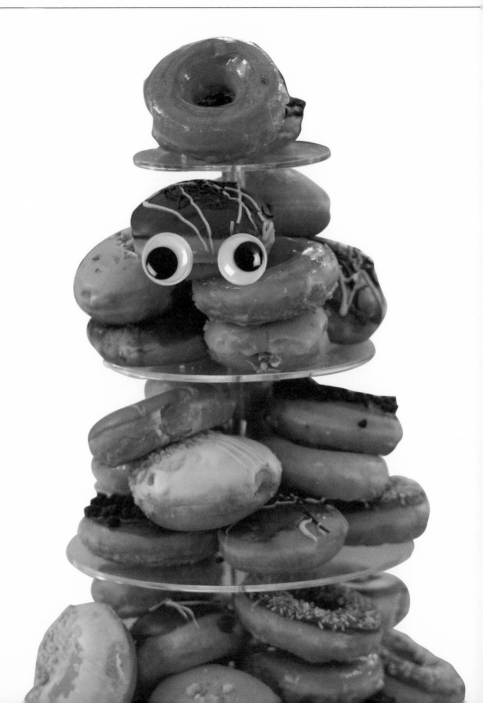

Eat according to your circadian rhythm.

—

Circadian rhythm (our brain clock) evolved over thousands of years to organize our cells into a day phase and a night phase. Eating during the day phase is biologically most effecient.

When we eat at night, our cells continue their daytime activities, neglecting important night-time recovery activities.

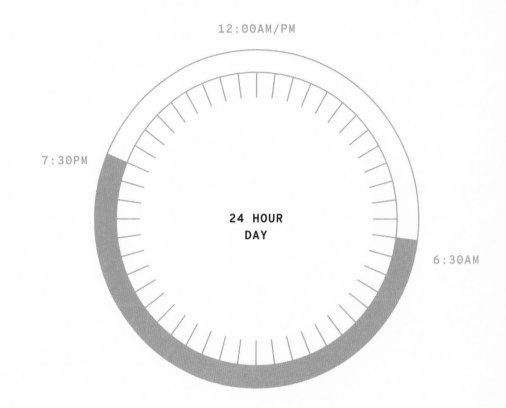

6:30AM

Day Phase Begins

By eating during the day, you allow your digestive system cells to process and absorb nutrients.

7:30PM

Night Phase Begins

If you avoid eating at night, you allow for a fasting period in which your cells eliminate waste and repair themselves.

Source: "Neurobiology of circadian rhythm regulation." Alan Rosenwasser, Fred Turek

And don't forget to make a toast and share a happy meal.

———

No, not that type of happy meal. You can make any meal a happy meal by sharing it with friends. Food, drink, and good company can add important psycho-social value to daily life.

Shared meals promote social bonding, cooperation, and relationship building.

Sources: "All in the family: Dinner tables linked to less obesity." Ellen Van Kleef,
"Knowing someone who is happy increases your likelihood of happiness by 15 percent." Framingham Heart Study

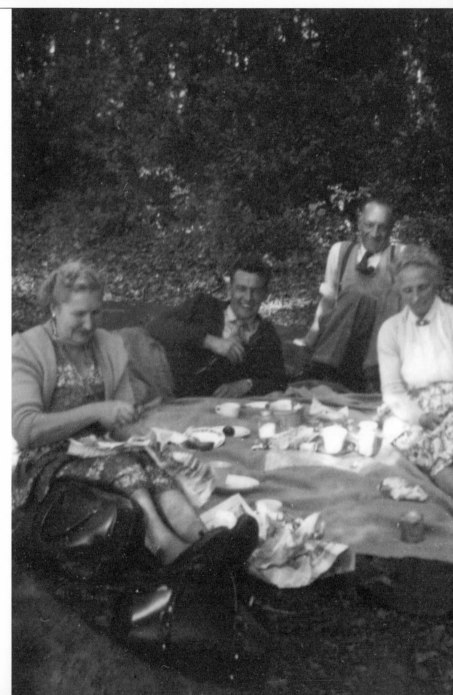

Exercise

Now let's talk about **exercise.**

—

The research is consistent and clear: exercise has a wide range of near- and long-term benefits. Regular excerise improves brain and physical performance, reduces anxiety, increases happiness, and increases lifespan.

On average, people spend roughly 9,000 hours of their life exercising (that's nearly 1 year).

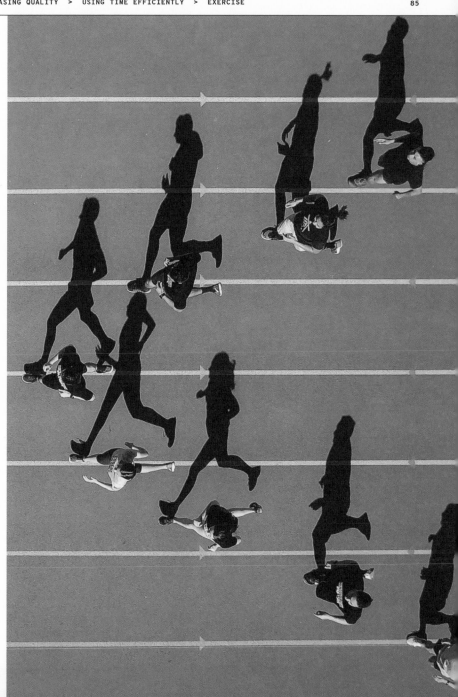

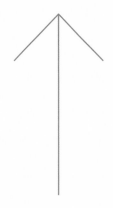

REGULAR EXCERISE
INCREASES

Cognition
Sleep
Digestive system health
Bone health
Physical function
Memory

The research is clear:
**you'd be foolish not to
exercise regularly.**

Exercise improves almost
all measures of health and
well-being.

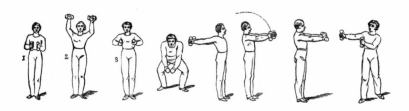

REGULAR EXCERISE
DECREASES

Obesity
Cardiovascular disease
Type-2 diabetes
Certain cancers
Dementia
Anxiety
Stress

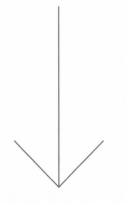

Source: "The anti- inflammatory effects of exercise: mechanisms and implications for the preventionand treatment of disease."
Gleeson, M., Bishop, N.C., Stensel, D.J., Lindley, M.R., Mastana, S.S., and Nimmo, M.A

Regular exercise increases your lifespan and gives you back even more extra time than you spend doing it (up to ~5 hrs/week).

Lifespan Increases with Physical Activity

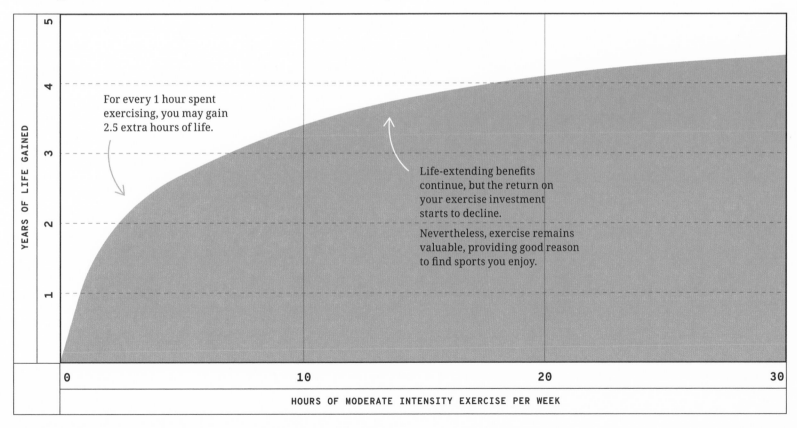

For every 1 hour spent exercising, you may gain 2.5 extra hours of life.

Life-extending benefits continue, but the return on your exercise investment starts to decline.

Nevertheless, exercise remains valuable, providing good reason to find sports you enjoy.

YEARS OF LIFE GAINED

HOURS OF MODERATE INTENSITY EXERCISE PER WEEK

Source: Harvard large scale research study; Moore, S., Patel, A., Matthews, C., Berrington de Gonzalez, A., Park, Y., Katki, H., . . . Khaw, Kay-tee. (2012).
Leisure Time Physical Activity of Moderate to Vigorous Intensity and Mortality: A Large Pooled Cohort Analysis (Physical Activity and Mortality). 9(11), E1001335.

4,000-8,000 steps per day significantly improves life expectancy, although 10,000+ steps a day is ideal.

Mortality Rates and Increased Daily Step Count

MEN   WOMEN

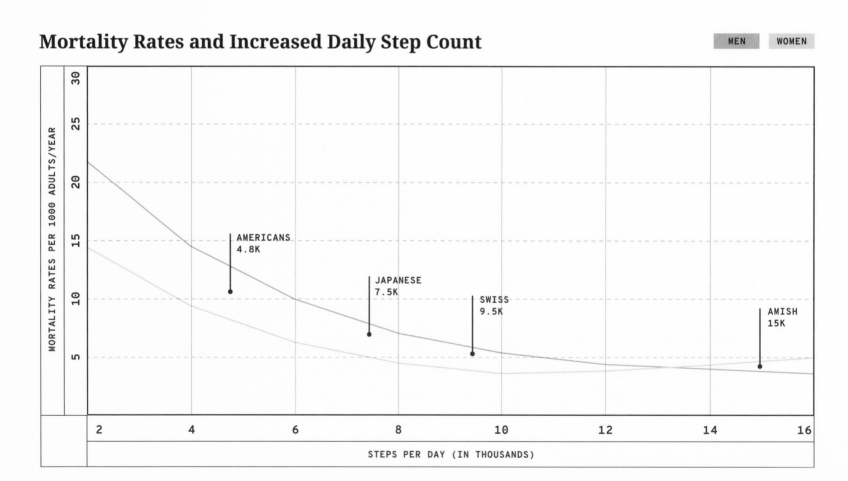

Source: Pedro F. Saint-Maurice, National Cancer Institute

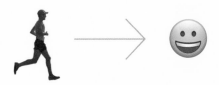

Exercise makes us happier, and it doesn't take much.

13 studies demonstrate the beneficial relationship between exercise and hapiness—with three main findings:

Even a small amount of exercise makes a difference in happiness.

1

People who exercise at least once a week report significant improvements in happiness in comparison to those who don't exercise at all.

Gains in happiness appear to reach a threshold.

2

Active individuals and very active individuals reported no differences in happiness levels.

No one type of exercise or intensity level is optimal.

3

Aerobic exercise and stretching/balancing exercises were equally effective in improving happiness.

Source: "A Systematic Review of the Relationship Between Physical Activity and Happiness." Zhang, Z., & Chen, W.

Aerobic exercise can take countless forms.

You have no good excuse: find an activity that suits you best.

———

Feel free to mix moderate and vigorous aerobic activities. A good rule of thumb is that 1 minute of vigorous-intensity activity is about the same as 2 minutes of moderate-intensity activity.

TYPE OF WORKOUT	ACTIVITIES
Moderate Intensity at least 2.5 hours a week	Walking briskly Recreational swimming Bicycling slower than 10mph Tennis (doubles) Active forms of yoga Ballroom or line dancing General yard work Home-repair work Water aerobics ...
Vigorous Intensity at least 1.25 hours a week	Jogging or running Swimming laps Tennis (singles) Vigorous dancing Bicycling faster than 10mph Hiking uphill or with a heavy pack High-intensity interval training Step aerobics Kickboxing ...

Feel your life getting longer?

Source: CDC

Add in some regular **muscle-strengthening**—and now we're really talking.

To maximize health benefits, the CDC recommends a mix of both aerobic and muscle-strengthening physical activities for adults.

Muscle-strengthening should be included two times or more a week. Focus on activities that are moderate or high intensity, such as resistance bands or weight lifting.

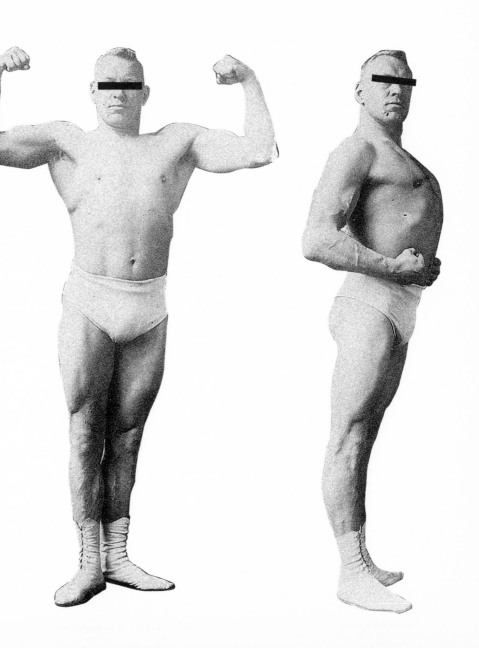

And for best results, **avoid eating right before exercise.**

—

If you eat too soon before exercising, you may inhibit your body's ability to burn fat for energy. Because your digestive organs and your skeletal muscles compete for blood flow, you may find exercise more difficult to perform.

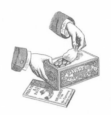

Snack

Wait at least 20 minutes before exercising.

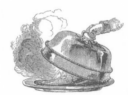

Small Meal

Wait 2 hours before exercising.

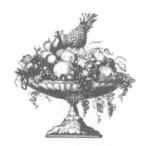

Large Meal

Wait at least 3 hours before exercising.

Source: "Does Fasted Cardio Provide Significant Benefits?" American Council on Exercise

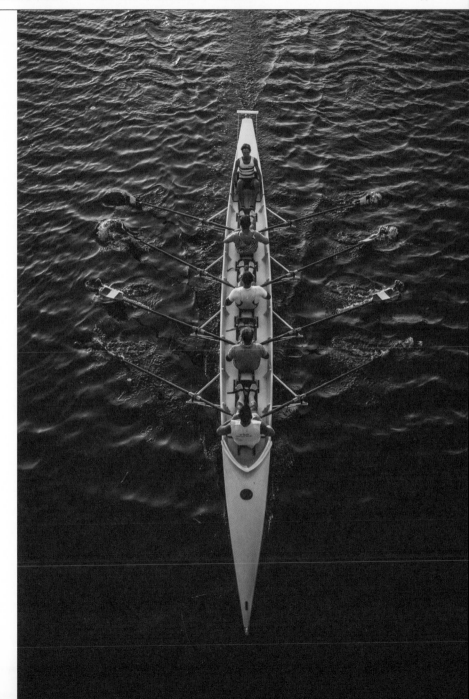

To really get the most out of your workout, **try exercising with other people.**

In one study, participants who exercised for 8 weeks reported enhanced happiness, reduced rates of depression, and improved overall health—especially after participating in group exercise.

Source: Gatab, T., & Pirhayti, S. (2012). The Effect of the Selected Exercise on Male Students' Happiness and Mental Health. Procedia - Social and Behavioral Sciences, 46, 2702-2705.

Motivation
- Overcome procrastination; the hardest part may be the simple act of starting or showing up.
- Know why you're doing it and remind yourself often.
- Set SMART goals: goals that are Specific, Measurable, Achievable, Realistic, and Timely.
- Find sources of intrinsic motivation.

Growth
- Growth comes from challenging yourself.
- Actively manage stress (on your body or in your mind).
- Learn and apply proper technique.
- Embrace "good pain" that makes you stronger.
- Avoid "bad pain" that signals excess.
- Give yourself permission to fail—so that you can discover what your limits are and what you can improve.
- Don't focus on competing with others. Focus on becoming better than you used to be.
- Don't give up. Extraordinary results come from extraordinary effort.
- Maintain a consistent effort over time, rather than sporadic bursts of effort.
- Allow yourself to rest and recover in order to perform your best.

Perspective
- Maintain a positive attitude and strengthen your resolve.
- Recognize your individual strengths and weaknesses.
- Identify interdependencies (e.g., sleep, diet, and stress level all impact performance).
- Share your highs and lows with others.

Once exercise becomes a part of your routine, you'll learn lessons that apply to your life more broadly.

Education & Work

Throughout our lives, if we're not at home we're probably at **school** or at **work.**

During our lifetime, we spend roughly 20,000 hours at school and 85,000 hours at work.

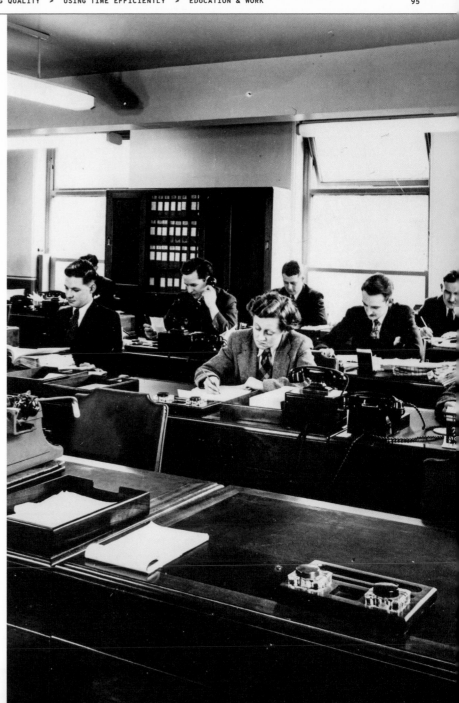

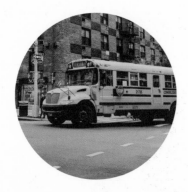

Before we get to work, **let's look at education.**

Many aspects of our current education system were built for a very different era.

	KEYS TO SUCCESS	WHAT REMAINS TODAY
Agricultural Era 1800s	• Hard work ethic • Summers in the field	• Traditional academic calendar (including summers off)
Industrial Era 1900s	• Standardization and interchangeable parts • Staying on task and keeping supervisors happy • 9 to 5 shifts • Emphasis on efficiency and correcting defects • Willingness to work in factory conditions	**Schools resemble factories in design:** • Centralized locations with standardized classrooms • Students seated in organized rows of desks **And are often run like them:** • Enforced schedules (e..g, switch at the bell) • Standardized testing • Age-based progression • Emphasis on producing results to be evaluated by instructor • Memorization of facts • Management to the average • Low instructor salaries
Digital Era 2000s onward	• Identification and application of unique strengths • Critical thinking based on first principles • Effective communication and teamwork • Creativity and self awareness • Strong STEM foundation • Ability to keep up with rapid change and automation	**But a few schools are innovating:** • Personalized and adaptive learning • Emphasis on finding and developing strengths • Encouragement of lifelong self-directed learning • Well-paid teachers evaluated on merit • Integration with technology • Frequent practice solving real-world problems with a team • Tailored teaching approaches (e.g., team learning, games, presentations)

The flow of progress is a human endeavor that takes time and effort.

Education plays a critical role.

HOW IDEAS BECOME PROGRESS

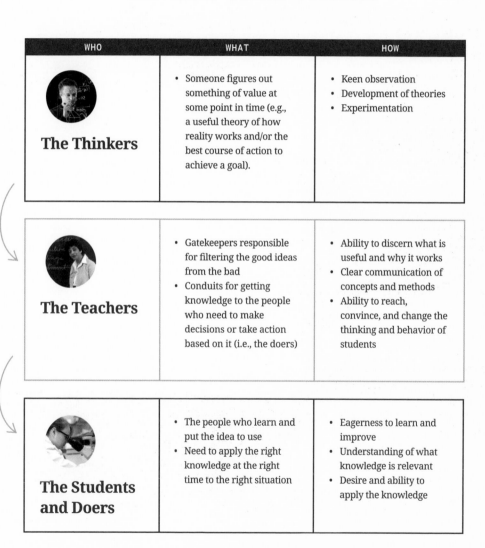

WHO	WHAT	HOW
The Thinkers	• Someone figures out something of value at some point in time (e.g., a useful theory of how reality works and/or the best course of action to achieve a goal).	• Keen observation • Development of theories • Experimentation
The Teachers	• Gatekeepers responsible for filtering the good ideas from the bad • Conduits for getting knowledge to the people who need to make decisions or take action based on it (i.e., the doers)	• Ability to discern what is useful and why it works • Clear communication of concepts and methods • Ability to reach, convince, and change the thinking and behavior of students
The Students and Doers	• The people who learn and put the idea to use • Need to apply the right knowledge at the right time to the right situation	• Eagerness to learn and improve • Understanding of what knowledge is relevant • Desire and ability to apply the knowledge

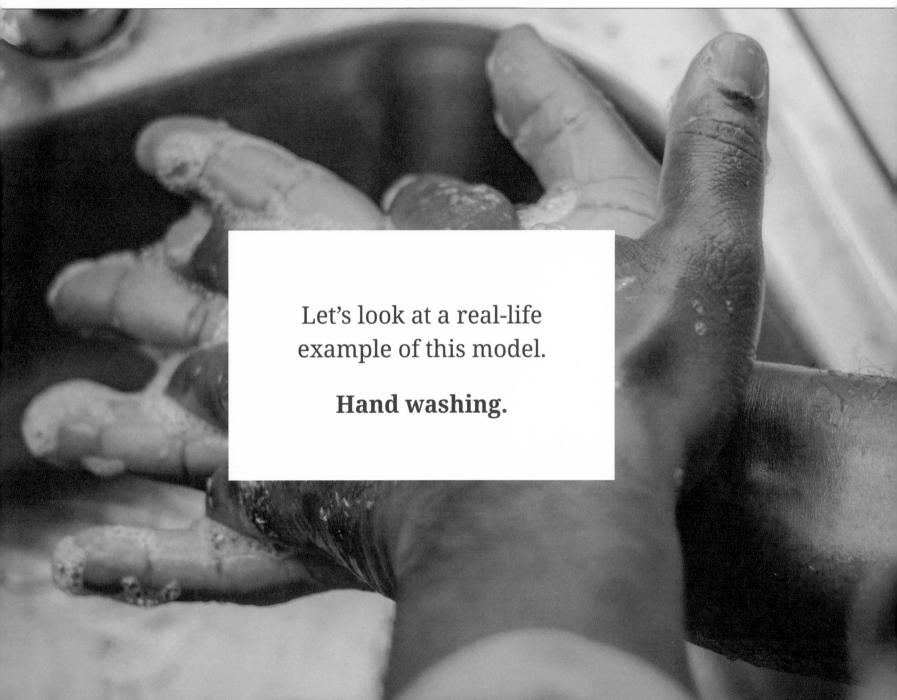

Let's look at a real-life
example of this model.

Hand washing.

HOW WASHING HANDS SAVED LIVES

For the world to accept the value of hand washing, it required years of education.

WHO	WHAT
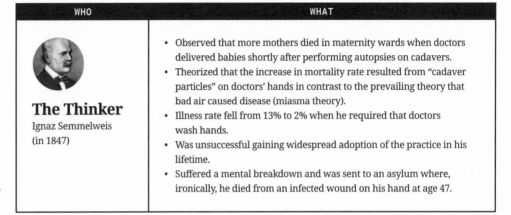 **The Thinker** Ignaz Semmelweis (in 1847)	• Observed that more mothers died in maternity wards when doctors delivered babies shortly after performing autopsies on cadavers. • Theorized that the increase in mortality rate resulted from "cadaver particles" on doctors' hands in contrast to the prevailing theory that bad air caused disease (miasma theory). • Illness rate fell from 13% to 2% when he required that doctors wash hands. • Was unsuccessful gaining widespread adoption of the practice in his lifetime. • Suffered a mental breakdown and was sent to an asylum where, ironically, he died from an infected wound on his hand at age 47.
The Teachers Doctors, Public Health Organizations	• Most doctors ridiculed the idea that they had a hand in killing patients. • Louis Pasteur develops germ theory, which becomes accepted in early 1900s. • Doctors slowly began to recognize the value of hand washing. • US Public Health Service (in 1961) creates a training video on hand washing for medical practitioners. • CDC (in 1975) publishes formal guidelines for hand washing.
The Doers Medical Practictioners, General Public	• Hospitals require doctors and nurses to wash their hands regularly. • More than one million people still die each year (~100K in the US) from becoming infected in hospitals. • Healthcare workers could prevent many of these infections by washing their hands effectively. • Members of the general public could avoid millions of sick days and additional deaths by washing their hands effectively.

Source: "It Took Surprisingly Long for Doctors to Figure Out the Benefits of Hand Washing." History.com

Education lasts forever, but school usually doesn't. When we're out of school, it's time to get to work.

Work can be great, terrible, or a mix of both.

Benefits of a healthy work life

- Personal growth and skill development
- Financial security
- Camaraderie and friendship from work colleagues
- A sense of purpose and mission
- Higher self-efficacy and confidence from competence on the job
- Potential for social impact through work

Consequences of an unhealthy work life

- Adverse effects on physical and mental health
- Unhealthy sleep schedule and diet
- Unhappy/stressful work conditions or commutes
- Lack of personal fulfillment or growth
- Unhappiness about compensation or benefits
- Stress overload from workload, performance, and job security
- Lack of social satisfaction
- Over-competitive work environment
- Poor relationship with superiors and colleagues
- Lack of boundaries with other spheres of your life
- Encroachment on leisure or family time

Finding the perfect job isn't easy.

Work represents a large portion of our time and identity. You're remarkably fortunate if you're able to find work that captures your interests, utilizes your skills, delivers impact, and pays well.

You may not find work that aligns all these features—but the more fulfilling you find your job, the better.

FINDING FULFILLING WORK

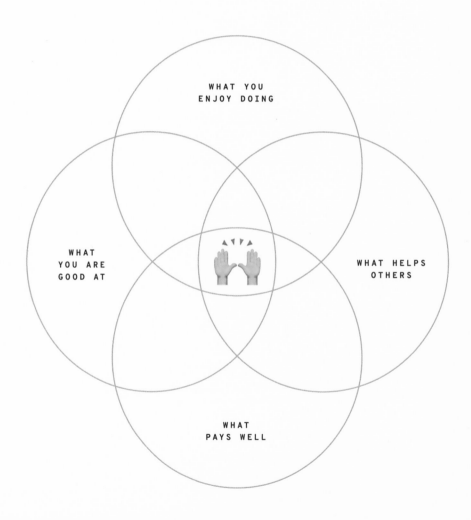

A lot of people think work sucks.

———

For every person who feels engaged at work, two feel miserable—and six more feel checked out.

Engagement levels differ regionally, with the highest rates of engagement in the United States and Canada (24%) and lowest in East Asia (6%).

What a missed opportunity for all. Engaged employees are measurably more productive and less likely to spread negativity.

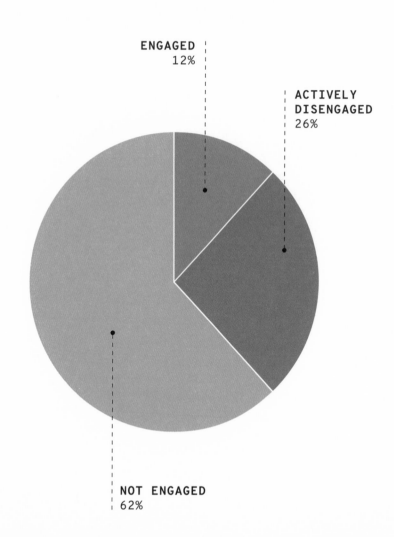

ENGAGED
12%

ACTIVELY
DISENGAGED
26%

NOT ENGAGED
62%

Source: Gallup poll of adults aged 18 and older in 142 countries, N = 150K+ 2009-2012

If you want to achieve your full potential, you'll need a growth mindset.

Your beliefs about your ability to change and grow can make a big difference in your career and life.

In one study, 40% of participants described themselves as having a growth mindset, 40% as having a fixed mindset, and 20% as unsure.

Frankly, you can develop new skills and interests. And you have the ability to change your mindset.

	Fixed Mindset	Growth Mindset
CORE BELIEF	Intelligence, interests, and talents are fixed at a set level	Intelligence, interests, and talents can be developed
WANTS	Approval To look smart	Desire to learn
RESPONSE TO CHALLENGES	Avoid them	Embrace them
VIEW OF EFFORT	Pointless or sign of failure	Necessary and the path to mastery
VIEW OF OTHERS' SUCCESS	Threatening	Inspiring
APPROACH TO FAILURE	Limit of your ability Gives up easily	Opportunity to grow Persists
TYPICAL OUTCOMES	Self-imposed limits (that become real) Hit a wall early Underachieve potential	Reach ever-higher levels of achievement Greater sense of freedom

Source: Dr. Carol Dweck, Stanford University https://www.psychologicalscience.org/observer/dweck-growth-mindsets

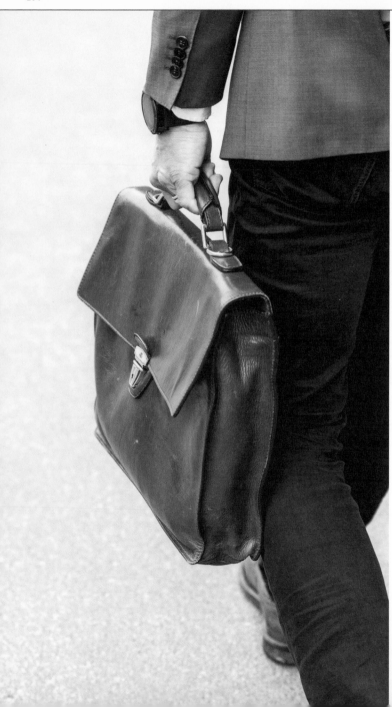

Ways to do better in the workplace

- Take advantage of available workplace wellness programs, which improve productivity and employee health.

- Have a positive outlook on your ability to complete work.

- Adopt a growth mindset, which can help develop persistence and expertise.

- Take your vacation days to help recharge. (Americans leave over 750M vacation days unused a year.)

- Take short, frequent breaks—and mix in exercise.

- Don't just sit there. Prolonged office motionlessness is linked with negative health outcomes.

- Take multiple short breaks rather than one long break.

- Participate in communal activities with colleagues (e.g., eating, drinking, socializing).

- Keep hydrated.

Kill your commute—or at least make it useful.

- Eliminate or reduce your commute by working from home part-time or full-time.

- Live closer to work (if possible).

- Make your commute less stressful by arriving to work at non-peak travel times.

- Use commute time for self-care and development. Find what works for you: audiobooks, podcasts, meditation, prayer, music, etc.

- Set tangible, achievable goals for your day.

- Modify your sleep schedule if you keep falling asleep during your commute.

Source: Stress that Doesn't Pay: The Commuting Paradox. Alois Stutzer, Bruno Frey

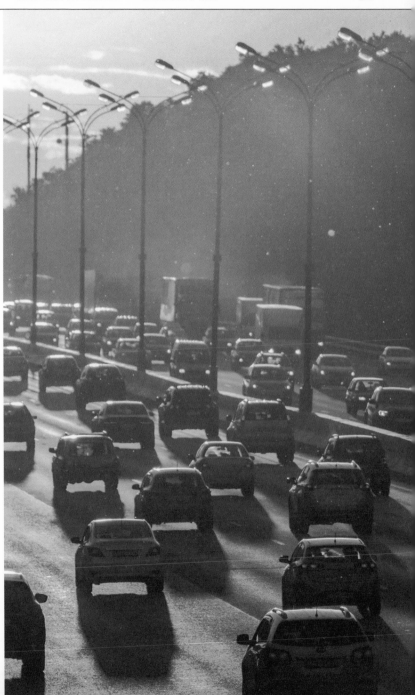

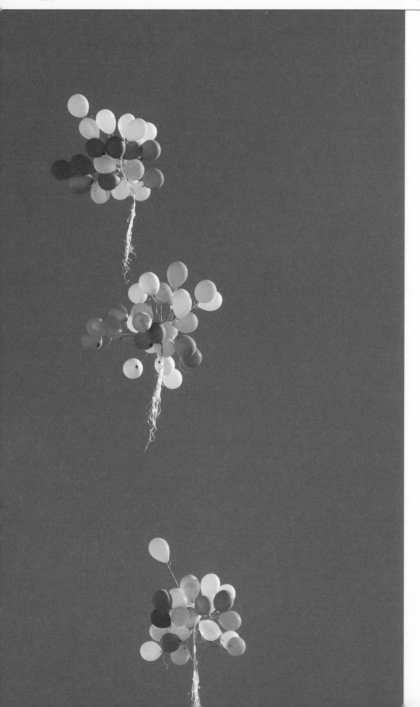

Take the time to unplug from work—literally and figuratively.

- Don't let work bleed into other spheres of life.

- Create "sacred time" away from work to focus on leisure, family, sleep, exercise, etc.

- Establish work hours, and try to avoid checking your work email outside those hours.

- Develop genuine relationships and interests outside of work.

- Plan for and go on getaways, both short and long.

Leisure & Vacation

After working hard, you deserve a break: **time for leisure and vacation.**

———

During our lifetime, we spend roughly 79,000 hours on lesiure and roughly 26,000 hours on vacation.

Characteristics of leisure time:
- Frequent or daily
- Home-based or local activities
- Usually built into a regular schedule

Characteristics of vacation time:
- Infrequent or sporadic
- Away from home and often requires travel
- Usually includes moderate to extensive planning

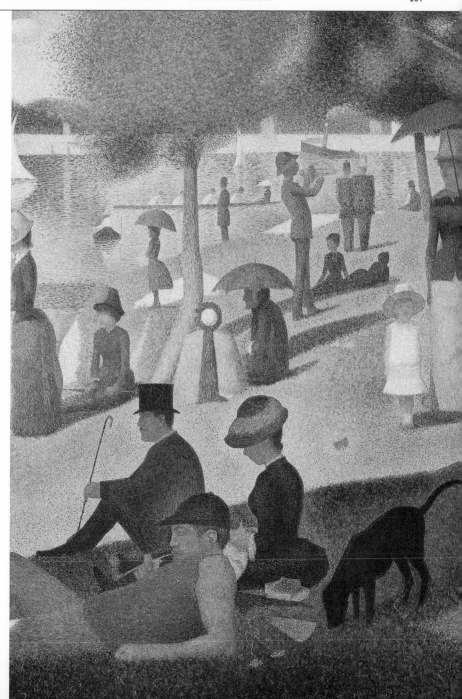

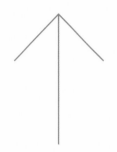

REGULAR LEISURE
INCREASES

Happiness
Cardiovascular health

Studies show that leisure improves physical and mental health.

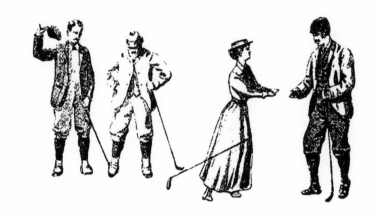

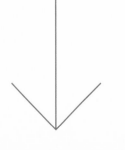

REGULAR LEISURE
DECREASES

Anxiety
Stress
Risky behavior
Substance use—and abuse

Not all leisure is created equal.

Healthy leisure is restorative and self-improving. Unhealthy leisure involves partaking in an activity to excessive levels, often to escape from (or tune out) reality.

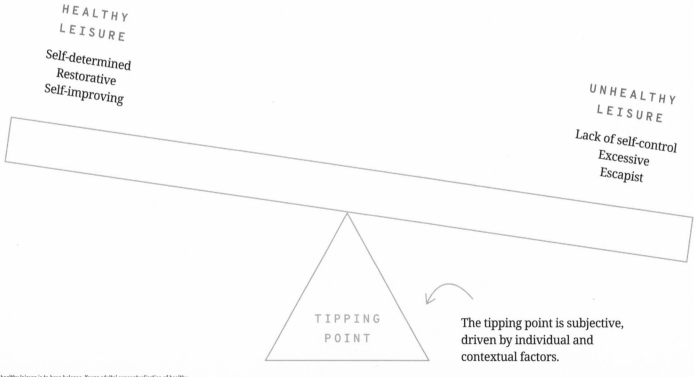

HEALTHY LEISURE

Self-determined
Restorative
Self-improving

UNHEALTHY LEISURE

Lack of self-control
Excessive
Escapist

TIPPING POINT

The tipping point is subjective, driven by individual and contextual factors.

Source: "To have healthy leisure is to have balance: Young adults' conceptualization of healthy and unhealthy leisure." Weybright, E., Son, J., & Caldwell, L. (2019). Journal of Leisure Research

KEEP HOURS AND
DAYS SIMPLE

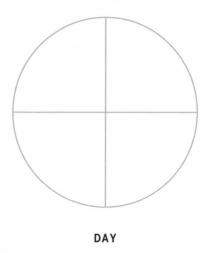

DAY

Variety is the spice of life—but be wary of multi-tasking.

———

Our day-to-day happiness depends, in part, on the variety of activities that we engage in.

Although we feel more stimulated (and therefore happier) when we fill longer time periods with more activities, we feel less productive (and therefore less happy) when we fill shorter time periods with more activities.

FILL YEARS AND
DECADES WITH VARIETY

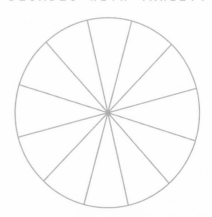

365 DAYS

Source: "Does Variety Among Activities Increase Happiness?" Etkin, J., & Mogilner, C. (2016). Journal of Consumer Research

Take time to reconnect with the great outdoors and those you love.

—

Spending time in nature promotes physical activity and mental health. Increased exposure to green space correlates with a marked decrease in mortality (8%–12%) from cardiovascular disease.

In a study at one hospital, patients whose room window provided a view of trees recovered a day faster—and reported less pain—than patients whose windows lacked a view of nature.

Explore nature together with family and friends. When we participate in activities with others, we help create intimacy, in part by providing each other with opportunities for supportive communication.

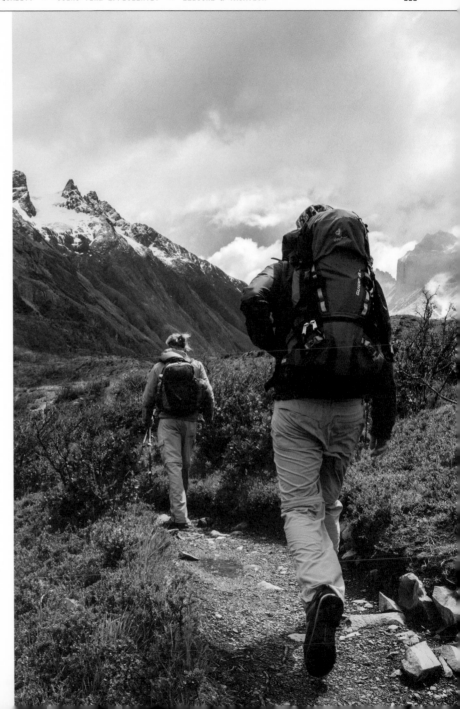

Ssources: "Nature in our lives: Examining the human need for nature relatedness as a basic psychological need." Hurly, J., & Walker, G. (2019). Journal of Leisure Research: Contemporary Trends and Issues, "How Nature Resets Our Minds and Bodies." The Atlantic

When you're ready for vacation, get your relaxation on—and seek new experiences.

___

Vacation provides the opportunity for:

1. Relaxation

2. Detachment from work

3. Mastery through experience (as you learn new things and gain new skills)

4. Personal control (as you decide what you want to do and experience)

Studies reveal that these benefits help decrease psychological and behavioral strain such as job-related stress, anxiety, and absenteeism.

Furthermore, one study found that people who vacation more frequently suffered fewer cardiovascular problems than those who vacation less often.

Source: "Tourism Experiences as a Stress Reliever: Examining the Effects of Tourism Recovery Experiences on Life Satisfaction." Chen, C., Petrick, J., & Shahvali, M. (2016). Journal of Travel Research

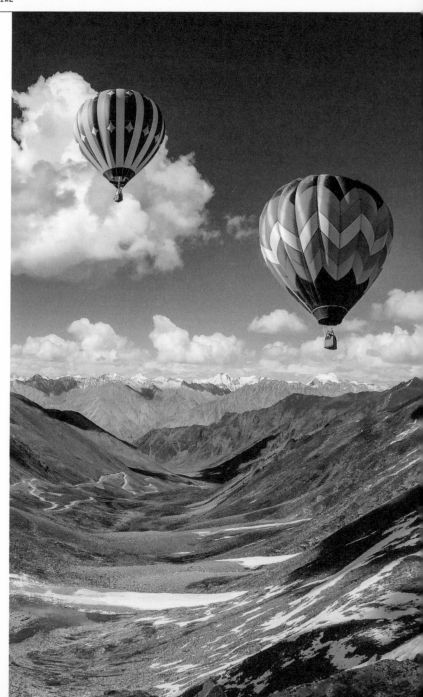

Vacation makes you happier, but
effects fade within 1-3 months.

Consider shorter and more frequent vacations.

Level of Life Satisfaction

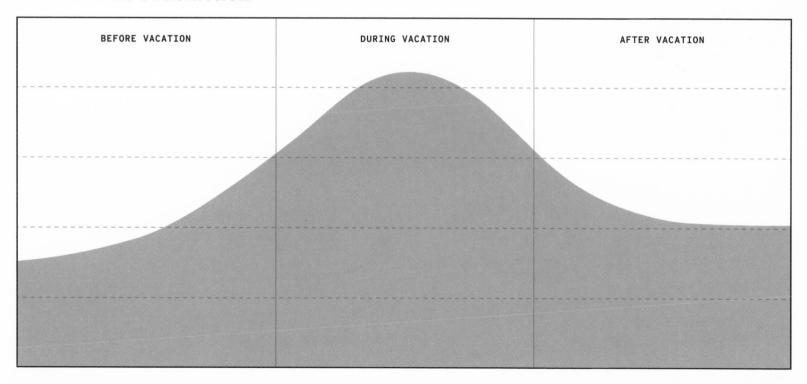

Source: "Health and Wellness Benefits of Travel Experiences: A Literature Review." Chen, C., & Petrick, J. (2013). Journal of Travel Research

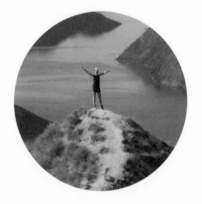

We remember the peaks and ends of experiences most— not the duration or average moments of the experience.

The peak-end rule is a psychological principle that suggests people judge an experience largely based on how they felt at its peak (i.e. its most intense point) and at its end, rather than based on the total sum or average of every moment of the experience.

A peak moment requires at least one of the four elements below, with the best having all four:

Elevation
Moments of happiness that transcend the normal course of events through sensory pleasures and surprise.

Pride
Moments that capture us at our best, whether it be moments of achievement or moments of courage.

Insight
Our eureka moments, which change our understanding of ourselves or the world and give us a moment of sobering clarity.

Connection
Moments that connect us to something beyond ourselves and are often social in nature (e.g., weddings).

Source: "Evaluations of pleasurable experiences: The peak-end rule." Amy Do, Alexander Rupert, and George Wolford

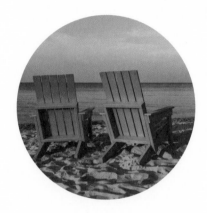

So again, don't worry if your vacation is a short one.

In comparision to shorter vacations, longer vacations don't produce longer-lasting memories.

A two-week vacation often produces similar positive memories as a one-week vacation, since we are often not forming diverse new memories with the additional time.

Recommendations:

- Consider incorporating tiny trips (shorter getaways) into your schedule.

- Avoid negative peaks or ends.

- Strive for positive peaks and ends. For example, take a mountain-bike trip with beautiful views (positive peaks) and treat yourself to a massage back at the hotel (positive end).

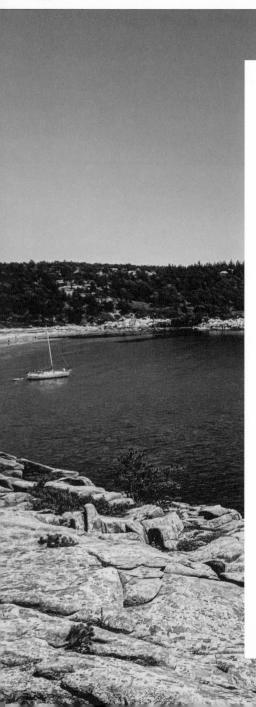

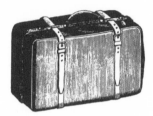

How to vacation

What To Do	• Eat healthy • Exercise • Get adequate sleep • Stay away from work • Decrease screen time • Learn something new • Have fun!
Where To Go	• Immerse yourself in the great outdoors. This promotes physical activity and mental health.
Who To Go With	• Share your vacation with family and friends in order to develop common memories and create intimacy.

Romance & Family

Devote the time to finding and maintaining a healthy relationship.

- People in committed relationships generally have lower cortisol (the stress hormone) and better mental health.

- People who are in love report feeling less physical pain.

- Married people demonstrate reduced risk of heart attacks.

- Romantic partners can improve their sleep quality by sleeping next to one another.

- Happy couples heal more quickly when administered blisters than singles who were given blisters (glad we weren't part of that study!).

- Partners tend to adopt each other's interests, viewpoints, and mannerisims. (So choose wisely.)

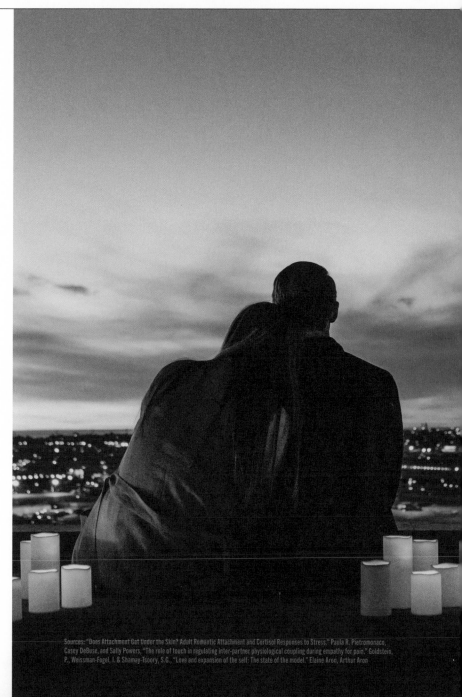

Sources: "Does Attachment Get Under the Skin? Adult Romantic Attachment and Cortisol Responses to Stress." Paula R. Pietromonaco, Casey DeBuse, and Sally Powers, "The role of touch in regulating inter-partner physiological coupling during empathy for pain." Goldstein, P., Weissman-Fogel, I. & Shamay-Tsoory, S.G., "Love and expansion of the self: The state of the model." Elaine Aron, Arthur Aron

First comes ~~love~~ education & career.

During the past 60 years, Americans have waited longer to get married.

Median Age of First Marriage in the United States (since 1890)

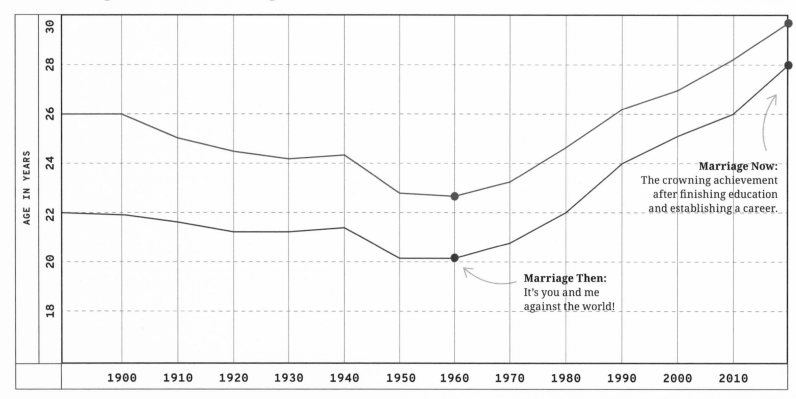

Marriage Now:
The crowning achievement after finishing education and establishing a career.

Marriage Then:
It's you and me against the world!

Source: U.S. Census Bureau

Roughly half of marriages end in divorce,
but marriage rates and divorce rates have
declined over the past 40 years.

Marriage and divorce rates in the US since 1890

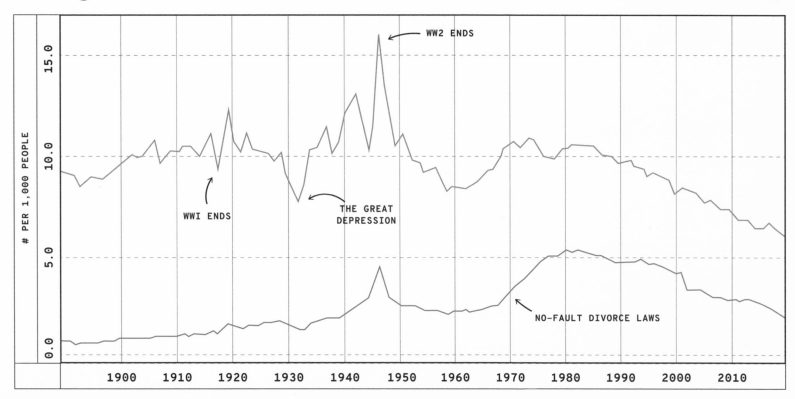

Source: "U.S. Marriage and Divorce Rates." Census Bureau

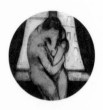

Keeping the romantic fire alive **requires both time and technique.**

Start and advance a relationship from a sense of purpose, not inertia
(e.g., don't slide into cohabitation, engagement, etc.—decide with purpose).

Maintain genuine relationships and interests outside of a romantic partner
(e.g., don't disappear from family and friends once you start a relationship).

Do things together that put the focus on something outside of the relationship (e.g., volunteering together).

Make time for couples based activities (e.g., playing board games together, which releases oxytocin).

Remain open, calm, and constructive when you communicate.

Clearly establish and respect physical, emotional, and temporal boundaries.

Be thoughtful in whatever ways you show affection.
- Physical touch
- Quality time
- Gift giving
- Acts of service
- Words of affirmation

Sources: "Sliding Versus Deciding: Inertia and the Premarital Cohabitation Effect." Stanley, S.M., Rhoades, G.K. and Markman, H.J. (2006),"Examining Couple Recreation and Oxytocin via the Ecology of Family Experiences Framework." Melton, K.K., Larson, M. and Boccia, M.L. (2019)

To save your future self time in therapy,
learn and apply effective conflict-resolution skills.

———

Conflicts are a natural part of any relationship.

When dealing with disagreements, use "I" statements rather than "You" statements (e.g., "I felt hurt when you..." rather than "You hurt me").

Don't exaggerate: avoid using words like "always" or "never."

Don't let grievances build: deal with them as they come up.

If a discussion gets too heated, ask for a time-out (with the promise of resuming the discussion).

Focus on the specific point of disagreement at hand.

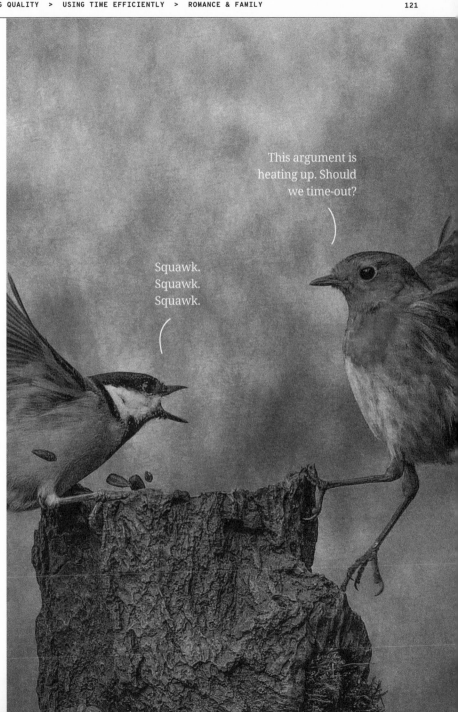

PROS OF HAVING KIDS	CONS OF HAVING KIDS
Get demoted from being #1 Having a child can make you less self-oriented and more focused on the needs of others.	**Crazy expensive** Average cost of raising a child in the US is $235K ...and that's before college.
Get to be a kid again Turns out that it's still fun to make snakes with Play-Doh.	**Environmental destruction** Having a kid ranks as the highest-impact decision you'll have on the environment (unless you cause an oil spill).
Become more invested in your community and the future You're likely to become more passionate about the quality of school systems and other social issues.	**Energy and time vampires** Kids are downright exhausting—and impact relationships, hobbies, and work. Your nights out will be numbered.
Experience new highs You will experience daily moments of joy and wonder in watching and helping your child grow.	**Reach new lows** From blowouts to tantrums to late-night fevers, you never envisioned your life quite like this.
Keep calm that a mini-you will carry on Take comfort that some part of you will carry on into the future (and hopefully visit you when you're old).	**Worry that they'll turn out alright** You may question your every move as a parent. Are you giving them enough attention? Too much?

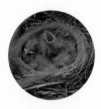

Bundles of joy. Sleepless nights.

Whether to have kids—and how many to have—are big decisions. Here are a few pros and cons.

Source: "The Cost of Raising a Child." US Department of Agriculture

During the past 50 years, the average number of children per family has **declined by half**.

A few contributing factors:

- Increased education
- Availability of contraceptives
- Advancement of women's rights
- Changes to economic situations
- Cultural shifts
- Lower child mortality rates

Children born around the world

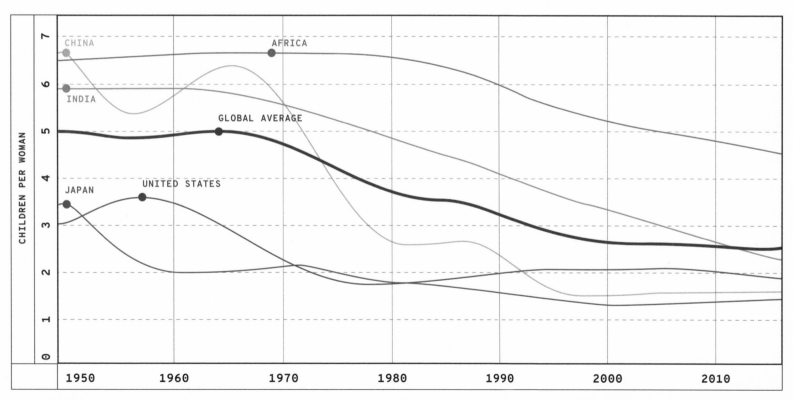

Source: UN Population Division (2017 Revision)

Now that we know how
to make the most of our
time, let's make sure we
have the most time.

Maximize Quantity

—

We all hope to live a long, healthy life. But nobody knows exactly when, or how, they will meet their eventual end. For "expert" advice on avoiding an early death, we can turn to two groups of people:

1. Doctors
Believe in science.
Practice modern medicine.
Advocate for healthy living.

2. Doomsday Preppers
Always keep survival top of mind.
Hope for the best—but prepare for the worst.

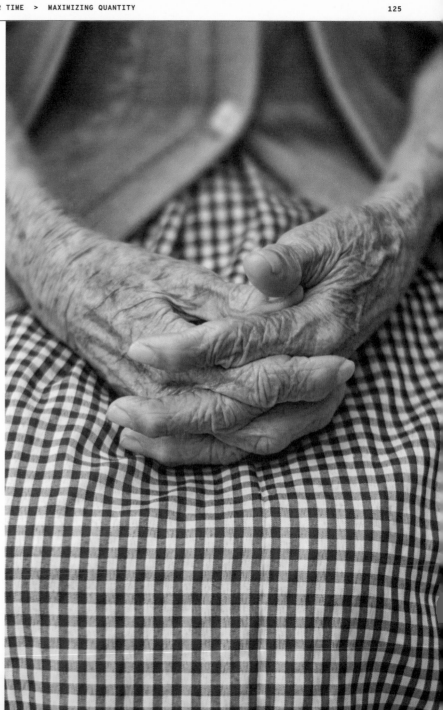

No one wants to die prematurely.

The thing is, our bodies betray us. (But let's be honest— too often we are the ones to blame.)

Global causes of death
(% of total deaths, 2016)

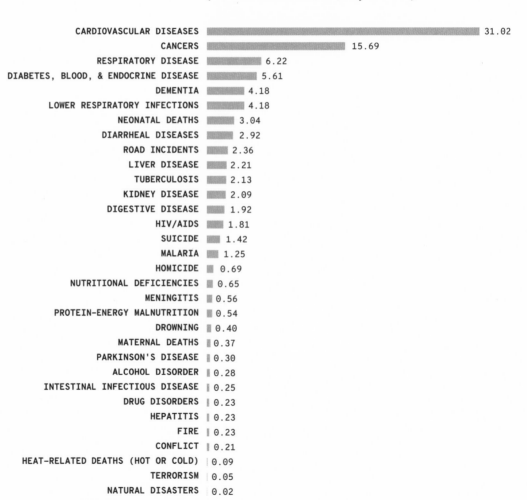

Cause	%
CARDIOVASCULAR DISEASES	31.02
CANCERS	15.69
RESPIRATORY DISEASE	6.22
DIABETES, BLOOD, & ENDOCRINE DISEASE	5.61
DEMENTIA	4.18
LOWER RESPIRATORY INFECTIONS	4.18
NEONATAL DEATHS	3.04
DIARRHEAL DISEASES	2.92
ROAD INCIDENTS	2.36
LIVER DISEASE	2.21
TUBERCULOSIS	2.13
KIDNEY DISEASE	2.09
DIGESTIVE DISEASE	1.92
HIV/AIDS	1.81
SUICIDE	1.42
MALARIA	1.25
HOMICIDE	0.69
NUTRITIONAL DEFICIENCIES	0.65
MENINGITIS	0.56
PROTEIN-ENERGY MALNUTRITION	0.54
DROWNING	0.40
MATERNAL DEATHS	0.37
PARKINSON'S DISEASE	0.30
ALCOHOL DISORDER	0.28
INTESTINAL INFECTIOUS DISEASE	0.25
DRUG DISORDERS	0.23
HEPATITIS	0.23
FIRE	0.23
CONFLICT	0.21
HEAT-RELATED DEATHS (HOT OR COLD)	0.09
TERRORISM	0.05
NATURAL DISASTERS	0.02

And over the course of our lives, risk levels change. We face a continually evolving gauntlet of tragedy.

% of all deaths by age

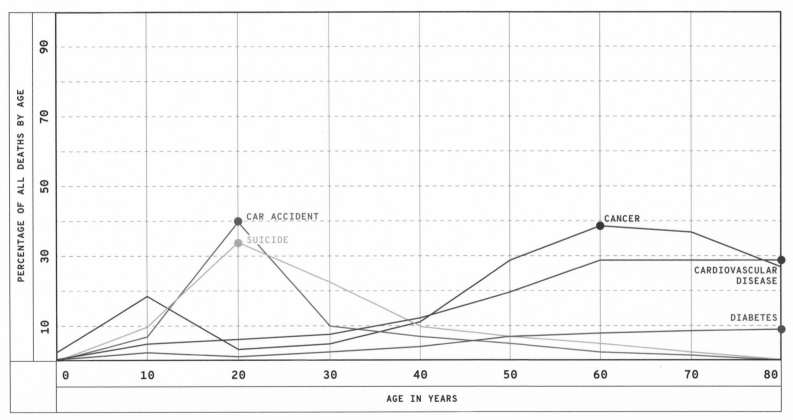

Source: National Center for Injury Prevention and Control, CDC

But we can maximize our lifespans in **several easy ways.**

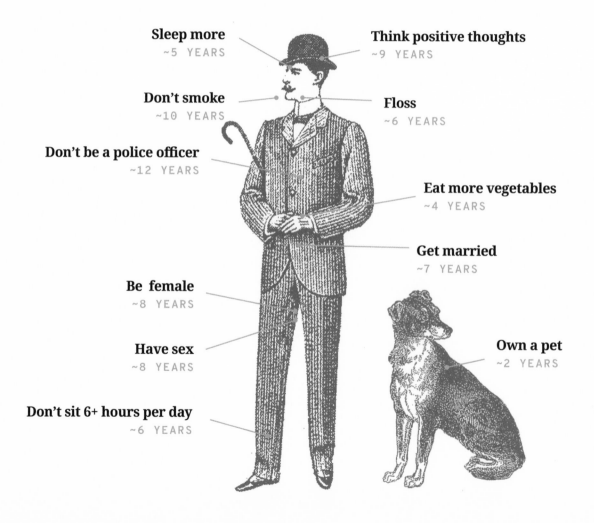

Sleep more
~5 YEARS

Think positive thoughts
~9 YEARS

Don't smoke
~10 YEARS

Floss
~6 YEARS

Don't be a police officer
~12 YEARS

Eat more vegetables
~4 YEARS

Get married
~7 YEARS

Be female
~8 YEARS

Own a pet
~2 YEARS

Have sex
~8 YEARS

Don't sit 6+ hours per day
~6 YEARS

Sources: "10 easy ways to lower your lifespan." Pleated-Jeans.com, "How to add years to your lifespan." DailyMail.co.uk, "The Health Consequences of Smoking." CDC , "Television viewing time and reduced life expectancy: a life table analysis", J Lennert Veerman, Genevieve N Healy, Linda J Cobiac, et al. 2011, "Life Expectancy in Police Officers: A Comparison with the U.S. General Population." John Violanti, "Dog ownership and the risk of cardiovascular disease and death – a nationwide cohort study." Mubanga, M., Byberg, L., Nowak, C. et al., "Does low meat consumption increase life expectancy in humans?" Singh PN, Sabaté J, Fraser GE

What can **doctors** teach us about maximizing lifespan?

1. First, do no harm.

2. Protect your body from chronic disease, which remains by far the greatest killer.

3. Establish healthy habits around sleep, exercise, and diet.

4. Get regular health check-ups to detect issues early.

5. Place a high priority on your health—don't wait until you're ill to take care of yourself.

6. Trust men and women of science rather than witchdoctors and snake-oil salesmen.

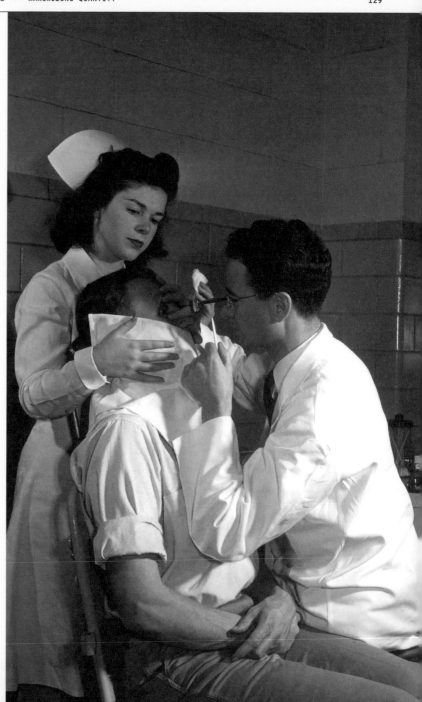

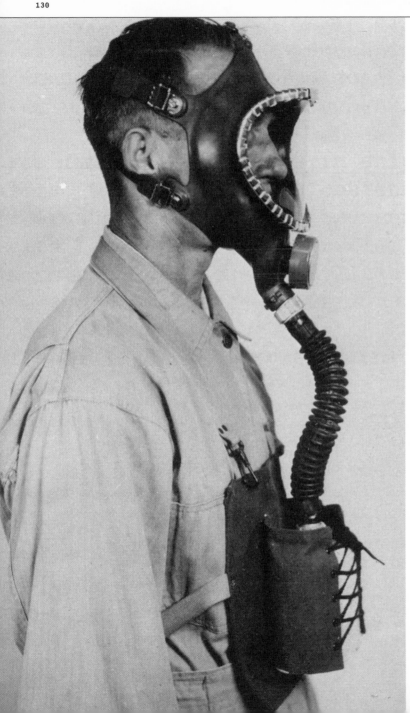

What can **doomsday preppers** teach us about maximizing lifespan?

1. Recognize that things aren't guaranteed to always keep getting better or even stay the same.

2. Stay alert: sh*t could hit the fan in a lot of ways.

3. Be prepared for a range of scenarios. Take action to be ready before a crisis.

4. Don't rely on others for the most important things.

5. Know what you need to survive and don't run out of those things (e.g. air, shelter, water, food).

6. Build redundancy into your preventative measures... just in case.

Still not sure how to maximize your time?
Try calling up **your grandma.**

1. Get some real-life stories.

2. Find out what worked for someone who is living proof of longevity.

3. Hear about how things were done in the good old days.

4. Make her day.

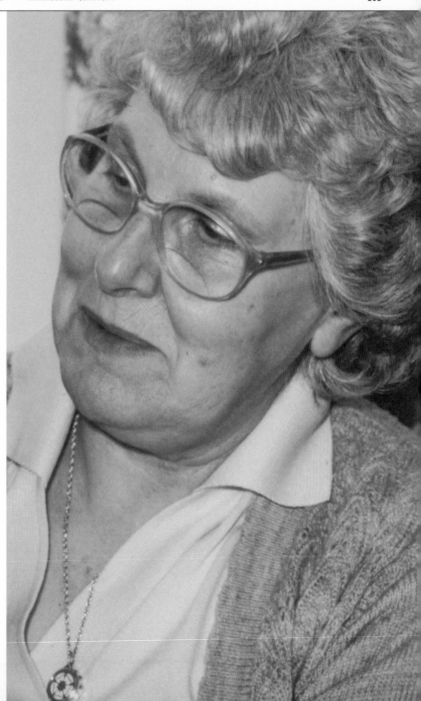

Finally, let's consider
how we **perceive** time.

Enhance Perception

———

Because everything we experience happens in
our head, we have a lot of power to enhance
our perception of time and life.

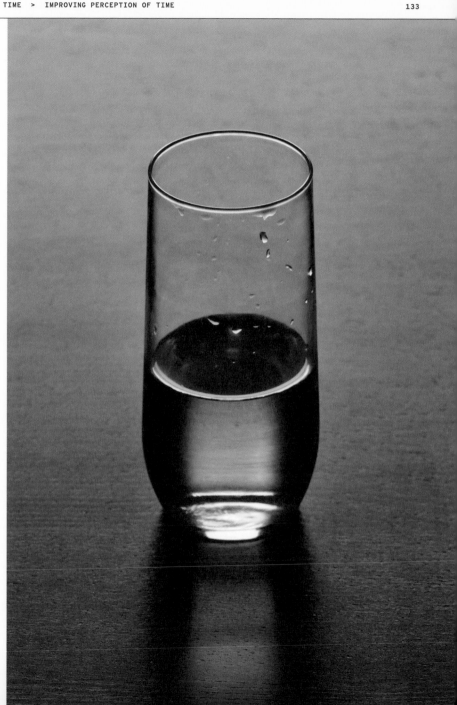

PHYSICIST

 NORMAL PERSON

Physicists think about time totally differently from how we experience time.

PHYSICIST	NORMAL PERSON
What is the difference between the past, present, and future? Unclear. Possibly all the same. The past and/or future may not even exist.	**What is the difference between the past, present, and future?** Past happened, present is nowish, and the future is ahead. They're distinct and different.
What changes the speed of time? The amount of gravity that is bending the fabric of space and time. Proximity to a source of mass and its density. The speed at which you are moving. Quantum things we don't understand.	**What changes the speed of time?** Things I do (e.g., sleeping vs. awake, busy vs. idle), how I'm feeling, and what's happening around me.
What time is it? Impossible to answer and nonsensical. Like asking what color is music. All relative depending on your position in the universe.	**What time is it?** Let me check my watch (or sundial).

HEALTHY WAYS TO CONTROL TIME

How we perceive the **flow of time** is highly subjective.

Our behaviors and circumstances can actually allow us to speed up or slow down time (in our heads at least).

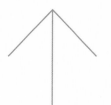

SPEED TIME UP

Flow state
Healthy stress
Older age and experience

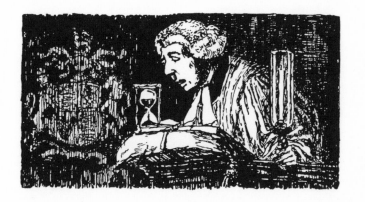

SLOW TIME DOWN

New experiences
Youth
Being in the moment
Feeling well rested

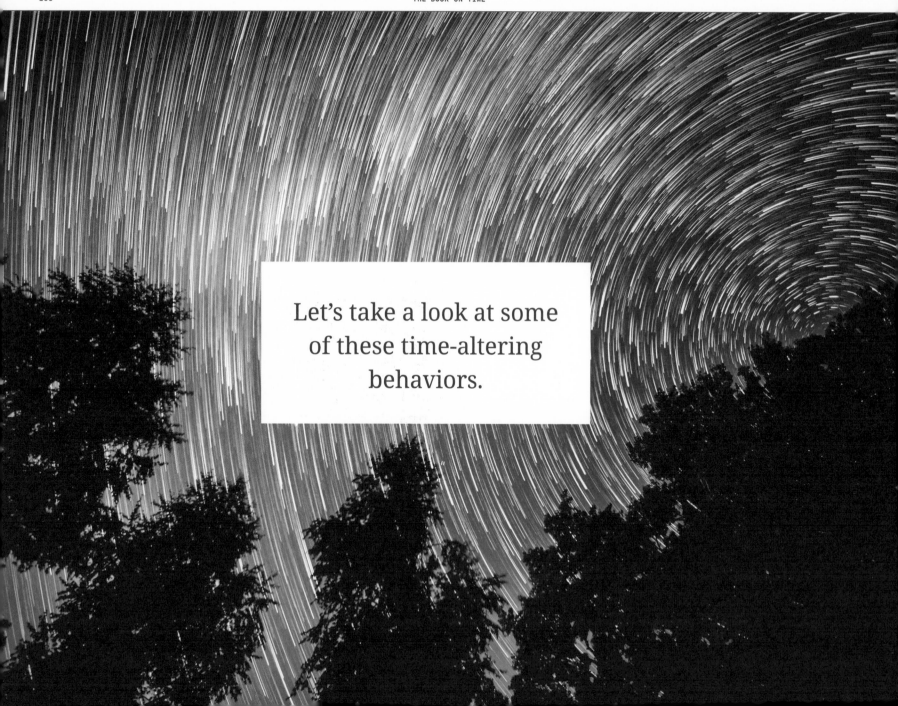

Let's take a look at some of these time-altering behaviors.

Experiencing new things
can make time slow down—and keeps things interesting.

—

When we experience something new, our perception of time slows down and our memories become more distinct. Time feels slower because our minds have to process and absorb more information and complex stimuli.

Novelty is often exciting and may lead to higher highs. But too many inputs can overwhelm us and lead to lower lows.

Routines can be helpful. They enable us to free up our intellectual resources for important and meaningful exploration in other areas of life.

Here's a reasonable way to approach life: **try anything once** (as long as it's not harmful).

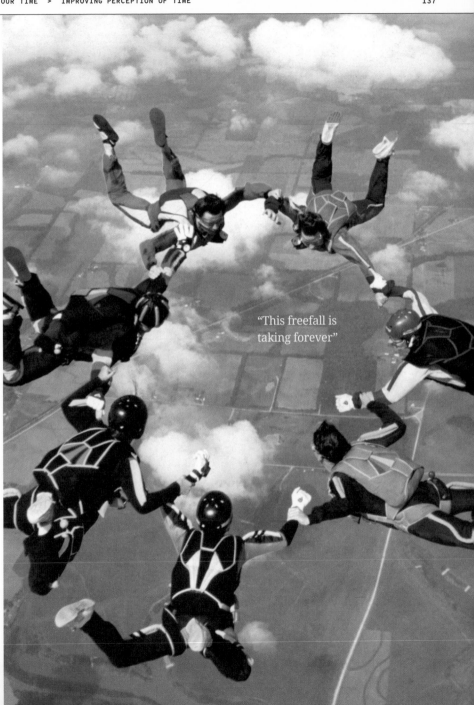

"This freefall is taking forever"

DIFFERENT STRATEGIES FOR NAVIGATING
NEW EXPERIENCES OVER TIME

■ NEW EXPERIENCE   □ REPEAT EXPERIENCE

Each of us has
different thresholds
for taking risks and
trying new things.

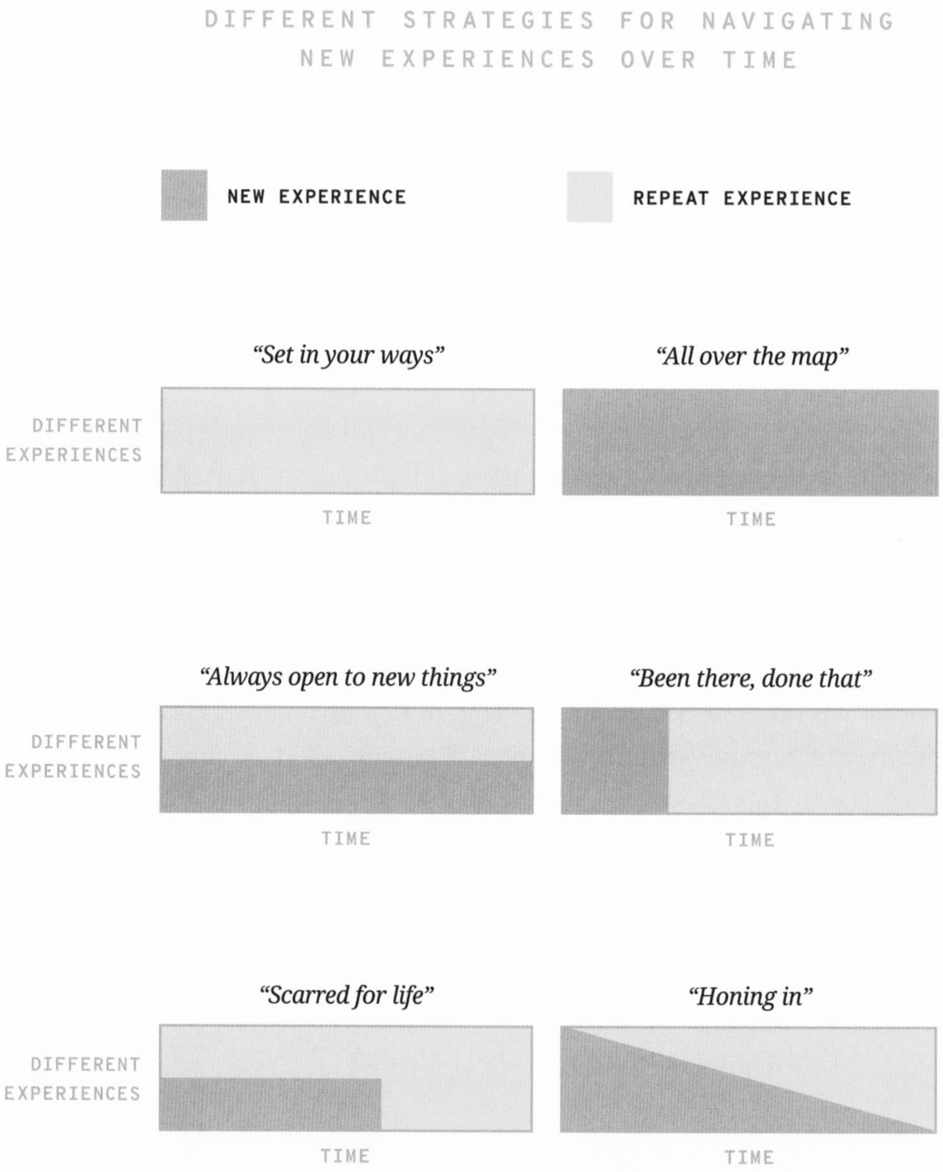

"Set in your ways"

DIFFERENT
EXPERIENCES

TIME

"All over the map"

TIME

"Always open to new things"

DIFFERENT
EXPERIENCES

TIME

"Been there, done that"

TIME

"Scarred for life"

DIFFERENT
EXPERIENCES

TIME

"Honing in"

TIME

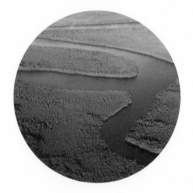

When you're in a **state of flow**, time seems to fly by.

But what's it all about?

What is flow?

Flow is the mental state in which we become fully immersed in what we are doing. It is characterized by heightened focus, full involvement, and a sense of achievement in the process of the activity.

What kinds of activities can bring the experience of flow?

We experience flow when we engage in controllable but challenging activities that require considerable skill, are intrinsically motivating, and deliver immediate rewards.

We increase the likelihood of experiencing flow when we choose tasks that align with our strengths.

What happens during flow?

While focusing on a task, we lose awareness of ourselves, but after we complete the task we strengthen our sense of self.

Our perception of time changes: hours pass in what seem to be minutes.

We concentrate fully: we become deeply and effortlessly involved in the task and transcend the worries and frustrations of everyday life.

Will flow improve our lives?

Yes! We are happiest and most fulfilled when we engage in absorbing activities that cause us to forget ourselves, lose track of time, and stop worrying.

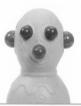

If you **embrace healthy stress**, time will really start moving.

———

Stress is simply the body's response to changes that create taxing demands. A little bit of stress is better than having no stress at all.

Rather than avoiding stress altogether, consider leaning into healthy stress.

Healthy Stress

- Motivates us, focuses energy
- Is short-term
- Is perceived as within our coping abilities
- Feels exciting
- Improves performance and leads to growth
- Helps motivate us to accomplish goals and ultimately find meaning in life

Distress

- Causes anxiety or concern
- Can be short- or long-term
- May appear to be beyond our coping abilities
- Feels unpleasant
- Decreases performance
- Can lead to mental and physical problems

We can also benefit by shifting
the way we think about stressful events.

"I'm so nervous and am going to fail."

"My pounding heart rate is freaking me out.
I can't think clearly..."

"I'm excited about this opportunity!"

"My fast heartbeat is my body's way of fueling
energy so that I can perform my best."

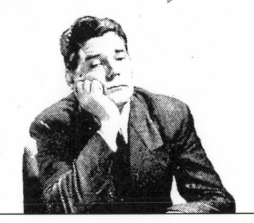

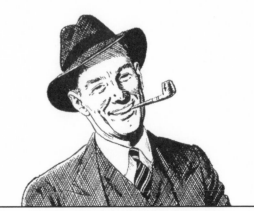

DON'T LET STRESS BECOME A THREAT

PERCEIVE IT AS A CHALLENGE

Source: Why time flies, Maximilian Kiener

No matter what, time feels like it's slipping away as we get older.

——

Time flies as we age, with each year representing a smaller fraction of our total experience. We lose the intensity of perception that we felt when we were younger. As the world becomes more familiar, we stop paying as much attention to the stimuli it provides.

Our brains also degrade. We take longer to process visual information via saccadic eye movements, and our production of mental images slows.

WHY CHILDHOOD MEMORIES REMAIN SO PROMINENT IN YOUR MIND

YEAR ONE

⊢————————————————————— YOUR WHOLE LIFE —————————————————————⊣

 When you're only a year old, one year represents 100% of everything you've experienced.

 When you're 30, one year represents 3% of everything you've experienced.

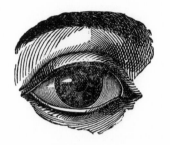

BEING RESTED AND IN THE MOMENT ARE
PHYSICAL AND MENTAL STATES

To slow down and savor time no matter how old you are, it's best to be **well rested** and **present in the moment**.

Well-rested
vs.
Fatigued

- When we're tired, we often lose track of time.
- Fatigue creates overlaps and pauses in saccadic eye movements that lead to crossed signals.
- Our tired brains can't transfer information effectively when we simultaneously try to see and make sense of visual information.

Being in the moment
vs.
Mindlessly distracted

- When we pay attention to the here and now, our brain absorbs and stores more new information.
- Active mental engagement is key.
- People who experience stress or depression may have trouble paying attention. As they ruminate about their problems, their minds wander and time feels like it is slipping by.

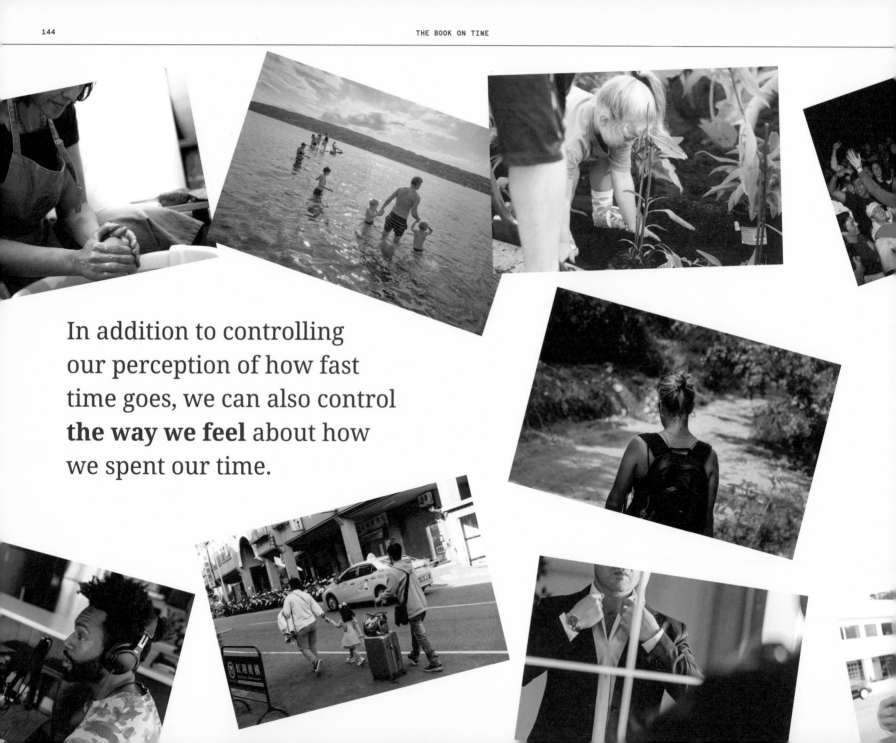

In addition to controlling our perception of how fast time goes, we can also control **the way we feel** about how we spent our time.

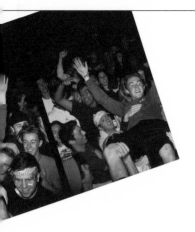

13 COMMON LIFE REGRETS

Many people look back with **deep regrets** about how they spent their limited time in life.

———

Significantly more deep-life regrets stem from what people fail to do (i.e., paths not taken) than from what they did in life.

LOSING PERSPECTIVE

1. Worrying excessively

2. Pursuing money as the primary goal

3. Not letting yourself be happier

NEGLECTING YOURSELF

4. Not prioritizing health

5. Living according to others' expectations

6. Over-indulging in alcohol and drugs

7. Falling into debt buying unnecessary things

8. Engaging in high risk behavior

NEGLECTING OTHERS

9. Prioritizing work over family and leisure

10. Losing touch with friends and family

MISSED OPPORTUNITIES

11. Not traveling more

12. Watching too much TV / being glued to phone

13. Passing up opportunities
(e.g., education, romantic, career)

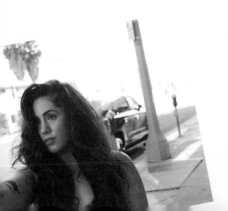

Sources: "The Ideal Road Not Taken: The Self-Discrepancies Involved in People's Most Enduring Regrets." Thomas Gilovich, Shai Davidai,
"Regrets of the Typical American: Findings From a Nationally Representative Sample." Mike Morrison, Neal Roese

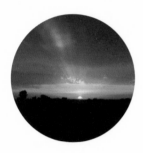

Here are effective ways to **avoid regrets**.

	WHAT HELPS
Be good to yourself	• Take frequent vacations • Invest in your health • Maintain positive self-esteem • Work towards financial security • Minimize worry and anxiety
Be kind to others	• Find a life partner • Spend quality time with family and friends • Forgive others • Volunteer and help others
Connect to something larger than yourself	• Practice religion and spirituality • Contribute to causes you find worthwhile • Experience nature
Keep it in perspective	• Cultivate and express gratitude • Find sense of purpose and meaning • Age gracefully • Value the limited time available to you • Keep expectations within reach • Find opportunities to smile—and laugh (you can even fake it until you feel it) • Focus on the best aspects of the past, present, and future

How we relate to the **past, present, and future** makes a big difference to our perceived well-being.

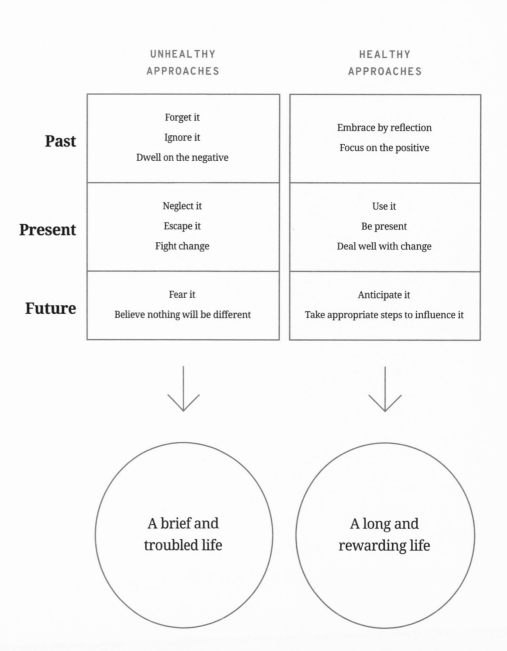

	UNHEALTHY APPROACHES	HEALTHY APPROACHES
Past	Forget it / Ignore it / Dwell on the negative	Embrace by reflection / Focus on the positive
Present	Neglect it / Escape it / Fight change	Use it / Be present / Deal well with change
Future	Fear it / Believe nothing will be different	Anticipate it / Take appropriate steps to influence it
	A brief and troubled life	A long and rewarding life

The day-to-day can bring us down.

Maintain a **larger perspective.**

———

Keep in mind that life is short, but don't get too caught up stressing about the lack of time in a day. One study found that when people were reminded of the scarcity of time in life, they found more enjoyment in life's ordinary pleasures, became more intentional in how they spent time, behaved more generously towards others, and felt time was more rewarding and fulfilling. However, when people were reminded of the scarcity of time in a day, they became less helpful to others, less physically active, more likely to shortchange other aspects of health (e.g., sleep, diet, friendships), and more stressed.

In our society, some people glamorize always being busy and view it as a status symbol. They may potray themselves as constantly busy to imply that they are more in demand, are more productive, and have more interesting things going on than others. In reality, people who are excessively busy may be just mismanaging their priorities and time.

It's easy to lose perspective. To get the most out of life, find space and time for reflection.

*"Life is short.
I better make the most of it."*

VS.

*"The day isn't long enough.
I'm stressing out!"*

Sources: "Research: Why Americans Are So Impressed by Busyness." Harvard Business Review,
"On the Psychology of Scarcity: When Reminders of Resource Scarcity Promote Selfish (and Generous) Behavior." Oxford Journals

And lastly, consider how to realign your expectations with reality.

It's sure to increase your happiness.

HOW TO INCREASE YOUR HAPPINESS

	WHAT TO DO
Reduce expectations	• Appreciate what you already have • Want less • Separate needs vs. wants • Reduce intensity of your desire • Change what you want • Give yourself more time to get what you want
Improve reality	• Better understand cause and effect relationships (i.e., drivers of your desired outcome) • Enhance your ability to influence outcomes • Build relationships with others who can help • Acquire the necessary resources
Deal well with the gaps	• Learn to accept reality • Focus on the positive • Invest more in things that are going well • Focus on things that are in your control—and don't stress the rest

PART FOUR

What are we trying to achieve—and how can we get it?

Pleasing Our Senses, Getting Along With Others, and Making Sense of the World

#lifegoals. Let's reflect.

You can get almost anything you want in life; but given the constraint of time, you can't get everything. Therefore, you need to figure out and prioritize which outcomes (i.e, goals) are most worthwhile.

Most goals stem from three universal and timeless human drives that start from birth:

- **Pleasing the senses**
- **Getting along with others**
- **Making sense of the world**

The better you do in these three domains, the more you will find enjoyment, love, and wisdom in life. Most suffering comes from problems involving how we think about, prioritize, and approach these three domains.

Ancient wisdom and modern science are converging on a number of effective strategies for each domain. Apply these insights in order to get the most out of your life.

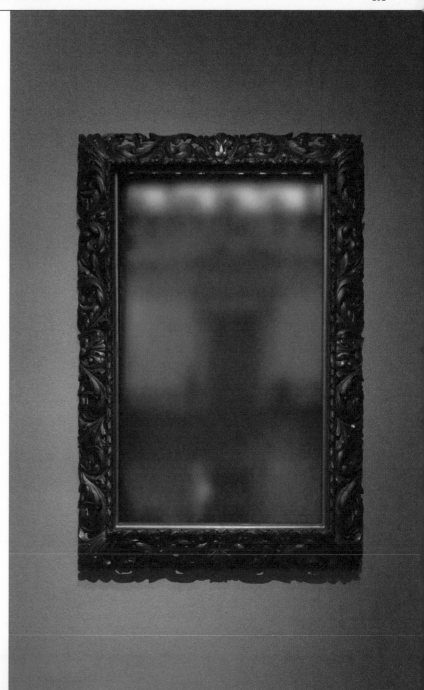

We all have the same **universal motivators.**

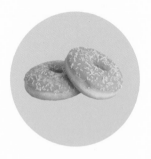

Pleasing our senses

———

I'M HAPPY IF...

I feel good and have moments of
physical and emotional joy.

I'M UNHAPPY IF...

I am in agonizing and/or constant pain.

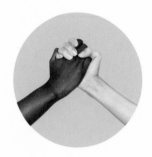

Getting along with others

———

I'M HAPPY IF...

People consistently treat me well with
respect and kindness.

I'M UNHAPPY IF...

People are cruel to me and unpredictable.

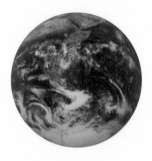

Making sense of the world

———

I'M HAPPY IF...

I understand why things happen,
can influence outcomes favorably, and
accept what I can't change.

I'M UNHAPPY IF...

Bad things that I can't control or
explain happen randomly to me and
people I care about.

Children start out entirely reliant on others until they start to make sense of the world.

UNIVERSAL MOTIVATOR	FROM A TODDLER'S WORLD...	...TO THE WORLD OF A CHILD AND BEYOND
Pleasing our senses	• Avoid potential threats to survival, such as hunger and cold • Enjoy milk, blankets, and naps • Become highly emotional when unpleasant things happen	• Learn to figure out how to get more of what you want and less of what you don't • Learn to regulate emotions
Getting along with others	• Communicate verbally (cries) & nonverbally (smiles) • Observe and imitate others • Depend on caregivers for survival	• Figure out which parent gives you what you want • Build (or lose) trust through repeated interactions • Learn to predict what people will be like
Making sense of the world	• Use play to test and refine mental models of how things work • Learn by observing and imitating others • Activate the imagination to create and explore possibilities	• Increase autonomy over time • Explore everything • Repeat what gets desired outcomes • Internalize others' behaviors and beliefs

Adults succeed by investing time in endeavors that provide enjoyment, love, and wisdom.

UNIVERSAL MOTIVATOR	ENDEAVORS	LINKED TO…	WHICH CAN PROVIDE…
Pleasing our senses	• Arts • Food & beverage • Recreation	• Senses • Pleasure/pain • Emotions • Appreciation	ENJOYMENT
Getting along with others	• Community • Religion • Government • Relationships	• Ethics • Culture • Morals • Empathy	LOVE
Making sense of the world	• Science • Education • Religion	• Logic • Meaning • Beliefs • Purpose	WISDOM

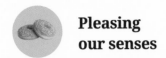

**Pleasing
our senses**

Embrace activities that stimulate multiple senses.

HOW WE EXPERIENCE DIFFERENT
ACTIVITIES THROUGH OUR SENSES

——

Food, nature, and physical activities stimulate many of the senses.

Screen time stimulates sight but neglects most of the other senses.

By slowing down and quieting your mind, you can meaningfully improve your awareness and enjoyment of different sensations.

By saying "cheers" and clinking glasses, we involve all 5 senses.

	SIGHT	SOUND	TOUCH	SMELL	TASTE
FOOD & BEVERAGE	●	•	●	●	●
NATURE	●	●	●	●	
SPORTS	●	●	●	•	
THEATRE & ARTS	●	●			
SCREEN TIME	●	•			

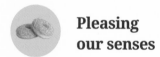 **Pleasing
our senses**

Manage your desires
so that they don't hurt you or others—now or in the future.

———

Our senses and emotional responses have been finely tuned over thousands of years in a world defined by scarcity.

In a world of plenty, we overdo instant-gratification activities, which may feel good but cause harm in the long term. 4 in 10 of all deaths are related to our inability to regulate our personal behavior.

Once you know which activities are harmful, you can respond in two ways:

Remove the temptation
(e.g., don't have junk food around the house, sell the gaming console)

Reduce the desire
(e.g., find alternatives, make being healthy part of your identity)

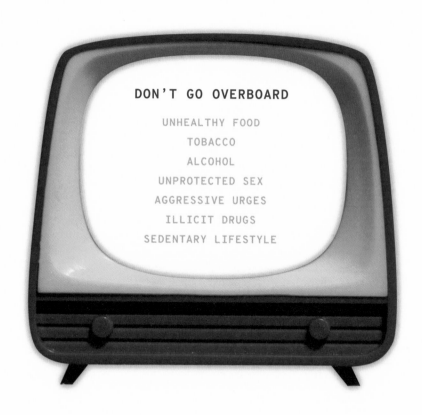

DON'T GO OVERBOARD

UNHEALTHY FOOD
TOBACCO
ALCOHOL
UNPROTECTED SEX
AGGRESSIVE URGES
ILLICIT DRUGS
SEDENTARY LIFESTYLE

Source: "Studies of premature mortality." New England Journal of Medicine.

**Getting along
with others**

Adopt a winning approach: focus less on yourself and more on others.

Be good to others. But don't just listen to us. (Who said it best?)

What is the essence of life? To serve others and to do good.

Aristotle

At the end of the day it's not about what you have or even what you've accomplished... it's about who you've lifted up, who you've made better. It's about what you've given back.

Denzel Washington

The best way to find yourself is to lose yourself in the service of others.

Ghandi

The unselfish effort to bring cheer to others will be the beginning of a happier life for ourselves.

Helen Keller

Volunteering is good for your health.

Harvard School of Public Health

Give and you shall receive.

Jesus

The meaning of life is to find your gift. The purpose of life is to give it away.

William Shakespeare

Life's most persistent and urgent question is, what are you doing for others?

Martin Luther King, Jr.

We make a living by what we get, but we make a life by what we give.

Winston Churchill

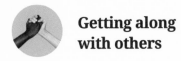

Getting along with others

Apply time-tested ways for getting along with others.

———

Think about how you would like to invest your time—and with whom.

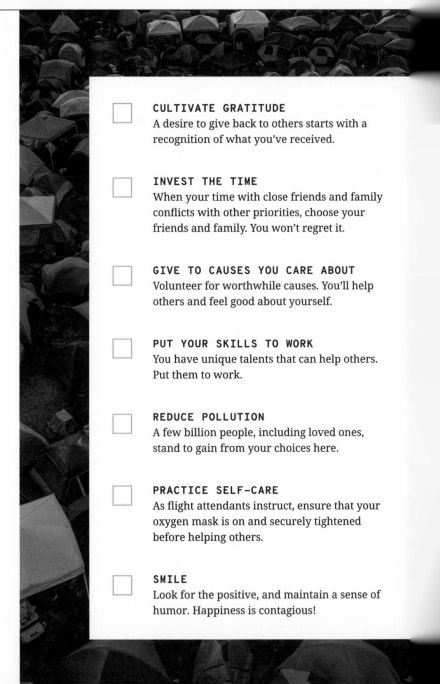

☐ **CULTIVATE GRATITUDE**
A desire to give back to others starts with a recognition of what you've received.

☐ **INVEST THE TIME**
When your time with close friends and family conflicts with other priorities, choose your friends and family. You won't regret it.

☐ **GIVE TO CAUSES YOU CARE ABOUT**
Volunteer for worthwhile causes. You'll help others and feel good about yourself.

☐ **PUT YOUR SKILLS TO WORK**
You have unique talents that can help others. Put them to work.

☐ **REDUCE POLLUTION**
A few billion people, including loved ones, stand to gain from your choices here.

☐ **PRACTICE SELF-CARE**
As flight attendants instruct, ensure that your oxygen mask is on and securely tightened before helping others.

☐ **SMILE**
Look for the positive, and maintain a sense of humor. Happiness is contagious!

Making sense of the world

Don't go it alone: accumulate wisdom by learning from others.

—

Identify the few things that you need to figure out for yourself—and learn most everything else from the experience of others.

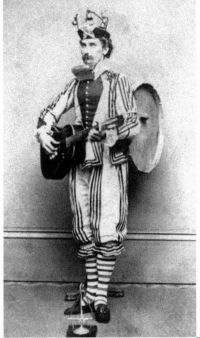

FIGURING THINGS OUT YOURSELF

FIGURING THINGS OUT YOURSELF

You need to figure out a few things for yourself:

- What questions in life are most important for you to answer
- What goals are most worthwhile for you to pursue
- How best to spend your time (and live your life)
- What knowledge you most need to succeed

To answer these questions, you need to look within. Allocate sufficient time and find the space to come up with a plan.

Because your answers may change over time, you need to deliberately revisit them periodically.

Remember that new experiences can help you expand and refine your understanding of yourself, others, and the world.

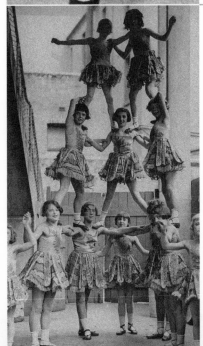

LEARNING FROM OTHERS

The secret to success in life is to repeat what works.

Learning from others is by far the best approach for most knowledge.

Some of the roughly 93 billion people who lived before you—or the roughly 8 billion people alive now—have already figured out a lot of what works, what doesn't, and why. Don't waste time reinventing the wheel.

If you encounter a particular challenge, you should be able to find others who can provide perspective and tactics to help you navigate successfully.

To learn well from others, be clear about what you're trying to learn—and seek those who know and can best articulate the answer.

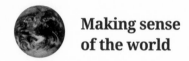 **Making sense of the world**

We live in an era of information overload.

Our brains can only process so much information at once (ever had to cram for an exam?)

For most of human history, knowledge in written form was scarce and hard to come by—until the past few centuries.

With the internet, we have an explosion of content not only in written form but also in audio, video, and other forms (e.g., VR/AR).

Our ability to navigate the modern world and make sound decisions depends on our ability to figure out what matters, what is true, and what to do about it.

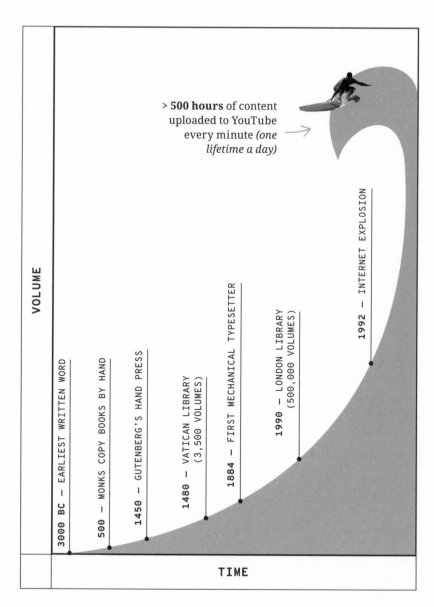

CONTENT GROWTH

> **500 hours** of content uploaded to YouTube every minute *(one lifetime a day)*

VOLUME

3000 BC — EARLIEST WRITTEN WORD

500 — MONKS COPY BOOKS BY HAND

1450 — GUTENBERG'S HAND PRESS

1480 — VATICAN LIBRARY (3,500 VOLUMES)

1884 — FIRST MECHANICAL TYPESETTER

1990 — LONDON LIBRARY (500,000 VOLUMES)

1992 — INTERNET EXPLOSION

TIME

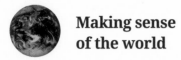 **Making sense
of the world**

Deal with information well— or end up with a scrambled brain.

———

Your approach to information determines whether you'll sink or swim in the information era.

DO
READ MORE (A LOT MORE) Reading is one of the most effective ways to transfer distilled knowledge from the brains of others to yours.
BE SELECTIVE Choose your information sources wisely. Forcus on those that are most useful and credible. Often these: • Have stood the test of time • Are sources you pay for • Provide a balanced viewpoint • Explain why and not just what
HAVE QUESTIONS Good questions serve as the filing cabinet for information in your brain. Without mental scaffolding to categorize and retrieve information you'll likely forget it.
PLAY IT BACK If you can't write down or explain the key points in a synthesized easy-to-understand form you don't understand it.
MAKE YOUR OWN LEARNING PLAN Be intentional about developing your wisdom. Identify what you want to know, where and when you'll look for the insight, and what you'll do with it.
DEVELOP A HABIT Build learning into your daily habits; knowledge accumulates over time.

DON'T
GET CAUGHT UP IN THE NEWS Be particularly wary of "free" sources that may have a slant.
TAKE THE BAIT If an information source often makes you feel strong emotions like anger, it's usually a sign you're being manipulated and not getting the full story.
BELIEVE EVERYTHING YOU READ We can't believe we have to say this (but we've just said it).
LET THE ALGORITHM BRING YOU DOWN We live in a time of infinite scrolling and continuous play. The machine learning and artificial intelligence that run these algorithms are optimized to make their owners more money, not make you wiser or happier.

PART FIVE

How can we navigate transitions successfully?

Dealing Well With Change

Dealing well with time means dealing well with **change.**

Time is a measure of change. If everything suddenly froze, nothing would change—and in theory time would stop. We can't stop time, nor can we stop change. Instead, we should expect change, prepare for it, and make the most of it.

We're not alone in experiencing change. Almost all of the changes and transitions that we encounter are experienced by others as well. Rather than rely exclusively on yourself to figure out the path through it, find out how others have navigated similar situations.

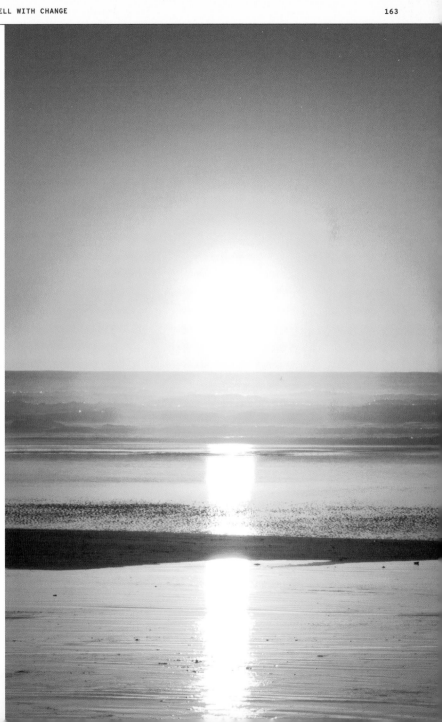

Our satisfaction with life is likely to change over time. Check out the "**Happiness U-Curve.**"

Overall Life Satisfaction, United Kingdom

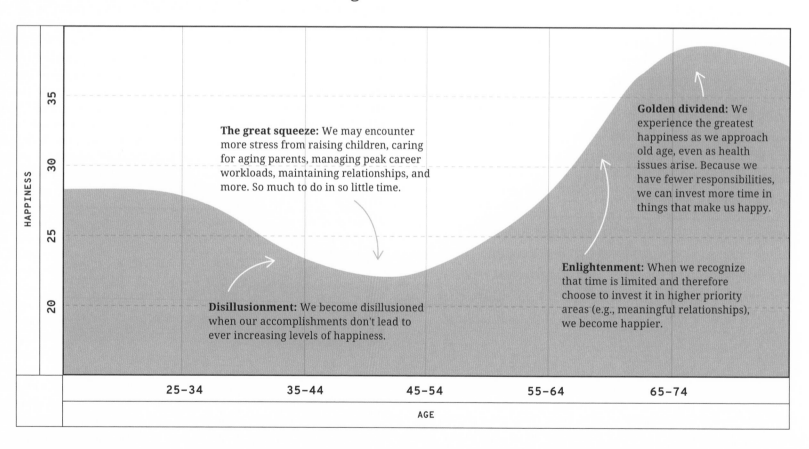

The great squeeze: We may encounter more stress from raising children, caring for aging parents, managing peak career workloads, maintaining relationships, and more. So much to do in so little time.

Golden dividend: We experience the greatest happiness as we approach old age, even as health issues arise. Because we have fewer responsibilities, we can invest more time in things that make us happy.

Disillusionment: We become disillusioned when our accomplishments don't lead to ever increasing levels of happiness.

Enlightenment: When we recognize that time is limited and therefore choose to invest it in higher priority areas (e.g., meaningful relationships), we become happier.

HAPPINESS

35
30
25
20

25–34   35–44   45–54   55–64   65–74

AGE

Source: UK Office of National Statistics

Throughout our lifetime, change happens **both internally and externally.**

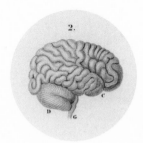

Internal Realizations

Internal changes may be gradual and barely noticeable or can be abrupt and jarring (e.g., mid-life crisis). Each of us needs to decide for ourselves which values, beliefs, and goals should endure vs. evolve.

Ideally, we find a balance that lets us stay true to ourselves while acknowledging and operating well within a changing reality. And remember that figuring out what we don't want can be as impactful as determining what we do.

CHANGES IN

VALUES
BELIEFS
UNDERSTANDING
PRIORITIES
GOALS
INFORMATION THAT YOU FOCUS ON
EMOTIONAL RESPONSES

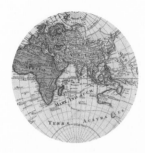

External Events

Everything around us is changing over time. Most change is predictable within a certain band of variability.

Occasionally, abrupt changes have a large impact. We can improve the quality of our lives by learning from prior events and preparing for future events.

CHANGES IN

ENVIRONMENT
ECONOMY
POLITICS
CULTURE
PERSONAL CIRCUMSTANCES
LIFE EVENTS / MILESTONES
LIVES OF OTHERS

Like all living things, we go through many small and large life transitions between birth and death.

We experience numerous transitions in life. Often, we experience increased anxiety around these transition periods. We typically find:

- Transitions are often most stressful during the first time we encounter them.

- A period of transition creates more uncertainty than a period of calm.

- Every transition requires us to adapt to new demands, which creates discomfort and stress.

We can be more or less effective as we respond to these transitions in search of a new normal. Although many of these milestones are new to us, others who have experienced them can provide advice on how to approach them.

"SEASONS" OF LIFE	COMMON MAJOR LIFE TRANSITIONS
Spring	• Greet the world at birth • Start a new school • Make new friends • Start a paying job • Begin first romance • Go to college/start vocation • Choose career
Summer	• Fall in love • Get married • Make major purchases (e.g., home) • Have kid(s) • Fail in big ways • Change jobs and careers • Succeed in important areas
Fall	• Hit a low point (e.g., divorce) • Achieve financial security • Encounter health scares (for you or loved ones) • Lose a parent (or parents) • Retire • Have grandchildren
Winter	• Focus on family and friends • Pursue hobbies and travel • Suffer from life-threatening illness • Fight for more time • Pass away

Don't let anxiety and worry rob you of your happiness or **waste your time**.

You can significantly increase both your effectiveness and happiness with a better organized mind.

We often avoid focusing on unpleasant things that may subconsciously cause us anxiety. When we force ourselves to confront a problem—and consider possible solutions—we almost always find that the problem becomes less scary and more manageable.

Find the right time to really examine what's bothering you—and explore what you can do about it. Once you have carefully thought things through, avoid revisiting or changing your mind unless you get relevant new information. Trust your insights and let them drive your decisions.

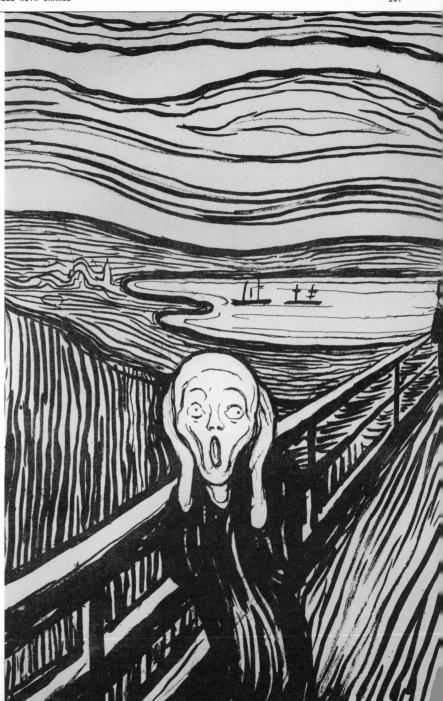

If you're worried and you know it, think it through.

APPROACHES WE CAN TAKE IN RESPONSE TO WORRY AND ANXIETY

ALL THE TIME
AT THE RIGHT TIME
SUFFICIENT THOUGHT
INSUFFICIENT THOUGHT
Exhaustion and burnout
Effective happy people
Chronic anxiety and worry
Missed opportunities

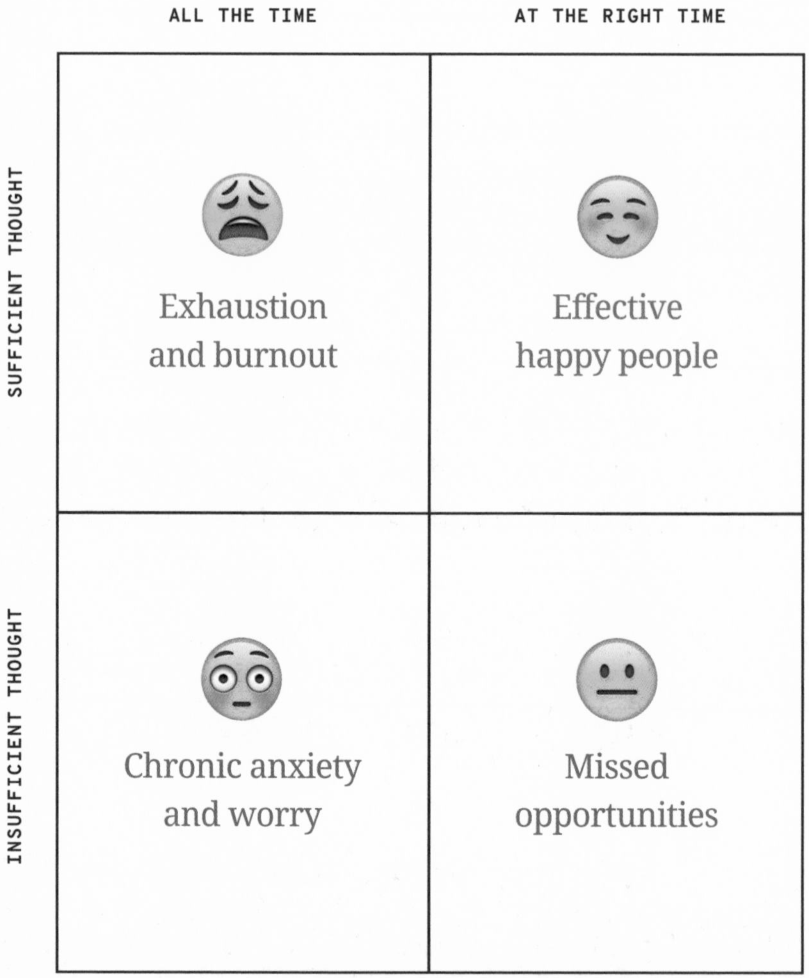

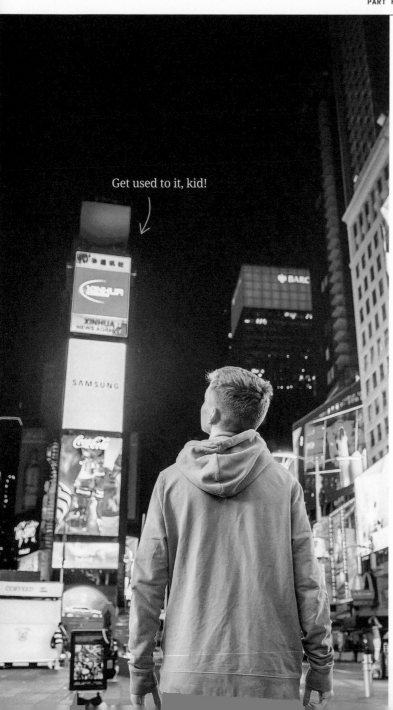

Get used to it, kid!

We've been taught to believe that **more** is always the answer.

Our consumption-centered culture has brainwashed us to believe that the solution to any problem—and that the path to the good life—is more.

Most of the roughly 3,000 ads per day that you were exposed to as a child—**and the roughly 6,000-10,000 ads a day that you are exposed to as an adult**—convey a common message:

- You would be more happy if you had more (sex, beauty, prestige, etc.)

- The reason you don't have more is because you are lacking something

- Compensate for your deficiencies (whether real or imagined) by buying more from us

When we fall for this three-part message, other people get what they want: they sell more products and make more money. But you are left with less money—and often less quality leisure time.

Paradoxically, by consuming less, we can gain more of the best things in life. (We often overlook or forget this truth because it's not exactly a profitable message to promote.)

Source: "Anywhere the Eye Can See, It's Likely to See an Ad." The New York Times

How, then, to get **more** out of life?
Embrace the light(ness) of having **less.**

	HAVING LESS...	...GETS YOU MORE
What you buy	• Physical possessions • Disposable things • Carbon footprint	• Money • Space (physically and mentally) • Better place to live (i.e., sustainability)
What you focus on	• Self-orientation • Anxiety and worry • Exposure to advertising	• Clarity • Focus • Happiness/contentment
What you do with your body	• Addictive substances • Processed foods • Sleep deficit	• Health • Longevity • Mental sharpness
How you spend your time	• Passive leisure • Mindless or excessive screen time • Exposure to toxic people • Constant hustle and busyness	• Meaning • Enjoyment • Wisdom • Well-being

PART SIX

What can we do to improve our legacy?

Making It Count

When you're gone, what will your great-grandkids think of you?

Do you know the names of your great grandparents? They're only three generations removed in a direct line that goes back roughly 10,000 generations to cavemen and cavewomen.

Your ancestors overcame many hardships and passed on their genetic code, values, culture, and knowledge— to help prepare you for the world you live in today. You're the living remainder—and reminder—of their legacy.

Do them proud—and be sure to leave something of value for the next generation.

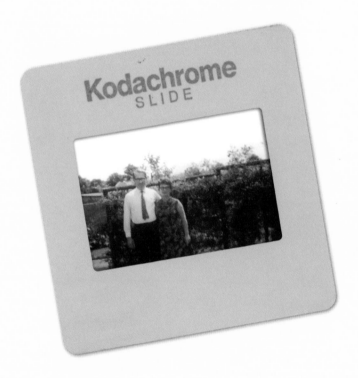

IMPACT ON OTHER PEOPLE	Distribution of your remaining possessions	1-15 YEARS
	Impact on everyone you knew	20-80 YEARS
	Organizations you contributed to	5-100 YEARS
	Written materials and digital footprint	INDEFINITE
	Children and their descendants	INDEFINITE

IMPACT ON THE ENVIRONMENT	Plastic waste	UP TO 500 YEARS
	Air pollution	UP TO 1,000 YEARS
	Changes to the physical landscapes	10-500 YEARS
	Other living species protected or destroyed	INDEFINITE

What will **your** legacy be?

Reminder of the big picture:
Earth has been around roughly 4,543,000,000 years[1],
and our human ancestors date back roughly 200,000
years. Our individual footprint on Earth may last
hardly any longer than a footstep in sand.

1 Based on carbon dating and convergence of other corresponding data

At the end of the day, your legacy is based on the impact you have on others and the world around you.

Very few things stand the test of time. Most of our thoughts, anxieties, and day-to-day hustle and bustle have little impact in the big picture of time, even in a few years from now.

Only two things are likely to endure:

- The impact you have on others and the world around you.

- Information that you create or pass on, whether it's genetic code, computer code, etc.

Give a bit of extra thought and attention to these areas in life. Don't wait until you're old before you consider what sort of legacy you want to leave behind.

To create an enduring legacy, focus less on yourself and more on the impact you want to have on the people and world around you.

Most of all, enjoy life, be kind to yourself and others, and keep in perspective the time of your life.

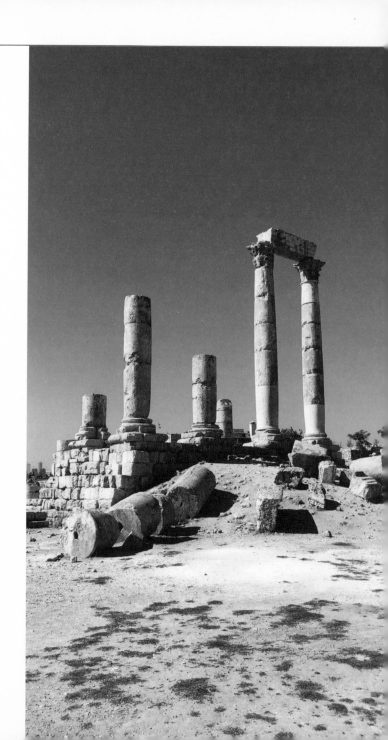

Putting it all in perspective.

⸺

Here are a few tools and tips for investing time well for a rewarding life and enduring legacy.

How to set priorities

- Regularly reflect on what you truly want in life—and why.
- Write a list of your goals in life. Prioritze and develop a plan for the most important goals. Review your plan periodically.
- Invest the time and effort to know yourself and better understand reality.
- Make a running list of things you enjoy and are good at (and those you aren't).
- Seek new experiences and knowledge.
- Find space and time to reflect on how you and the world around you are changing, especially during times of transition.
- Be intentional about your impact on others and how you can help.

How to make decisions

- For any potentially life-changing decision that you're considering, imagine that you're 80 years old in a rocking chair looking back on this decision. Will you be happy with the path that you are choosing now?
- Write down what your goals are, what possible paths are available, why some are more or less attractive than others, and what will likely ensue from each one. Pursue the best path. (Later, look back to see if the path you picked turned out as expected, and refine your thinking accordingly.)
- Consider what advice you would provide to a good friend faced with the same decision.

How to tell if you're doing it right

- Ask yourself, "Did I wake up excited for today? Why or why not?" What changes can you make so that you wake up tomorrow looking forward to the day ahead?
- When you sit still or meditate, do racing thoughts take over, or do you find yourself calm and at peace?
- Write the obituary you want—and the one you don't. Evaluate whether you are spending your time in ways that will lead to the the desired one.

Closing
Thoughts

—

If you're reading this, you have the most valuable asset of all: time. You also have the challenge of figuring out what to do with your remaining time. Will you waste it, spend it, or invest it—and to what end?

My hope is that The Book on Time helps you develop greater clarity and conviction as you think through these and other important questions for yourself. I also hope that you take away useful insights to improve your quality, quantity, and perception of time. The better the decisions you make impacting these three areas, the greater the benefit to yourself, others, and the world around you.

Finally, and perhaps most importantly, I hope that you will use your precious leisure time well. Not as unproductive time during which to mindlessly vegetate—but as time to pursue and experience the best of life. You'll have few life regrets if you use your leisure time in ways that reliably produce enjoyment, love, and wisdom. Because Emily Bernard and I believe that your leisure time is so important, we founded Bernard & Hawkes to help you and others make the most of it.

I wish you well and hope to see you on the journey.

About
the Author

—

ETHAN HAWKES grew up in a log cabin in Woodstock, Vermont. He came to appreciate the philosophy that "life is service" as a student at The Hotel School at Cornell University. As a consultant at McKinsey & Company, he advised on travel and customer experience topics. More recently, Ethan co-founded PlacePass and Bernard & Hawkes, with a mission of helping people spend time in more meaningful and rewarding ways.

Ethan loves ideas, people, and places—and seeks to fill his time with the best of them. In his leisure time, Ethan particularly enjoys taking tiny trips around New England with his family, especially if he can get out on a motorcycle, bike, or kayak. He has few regrets so far and would like to keep it that way.

Credits

DESIGN

Magnifico

Magnifico is a friendly design studio located in the coastal community of Newburyport, MA. They spend their time makings nice things for good people.

RESEARCH ASSISTANCE

Maria Jose Acosta, Jonathan Suh, and Hayoung Ahn

These talented Harvard University graduates majoring in humanities, economics, and neuroscience read and helped synthesize over 250 peer-reviewed academic studies (so you don't have to).

PARTICULAR THANKS

Becky and Jim Morgan—for their incredible support and example to others.

Don Berth, Rob Kwortnik, Kevin Speicher, and Nick Semaca—for their mentorship and encouragement.

Craig Snow—for editing expertise and setting the bar high.

The Hawkes, Wolfe, and Ramsey families—for role modeling the right values and priorities.

Caitlynn Ramsey and Everett Hawkes—for love, inspiration, and keeping it spicy.

Emily Bernard—for being an exceptional co-founder and person.

SPECIAL THANKS

To all who generously share their time and wisdom—thank you!

bernard & hawkes

We'd love to hear from you.
bernardandhawkes.com